Long-Term Care and Medicare Policy

Long-Term Care and Medicare Policy

Can We Improve the Continuity of Care?

David Blumenthal
Marilyn Moon
Mark Warshawsky
Cristina Boccuti
Editors

NATIONAL ACADEMY OF SOCIAL INSURANCE
Washington, D.C.

Long-Term Care and Medicare Policy: Can We Improve the Continuity of Care?
may be ordered from:

BROOKINGS INSTITUTION PRESS
1775 Massachusetts Avenue, N.W.
Washington, D.C. 20036
Tel.:   1-800/275-1447
          202/797-6258
Fax: 202/797-6004
Internet: www.brookings.edu

Library of Congress Cataloging-in-Publication data

Blumenthal, David, 1948–
   Long-term care and medicare policy : can we improve the continuity of care? /
David Blumenthal, Marilyn Moon, Mark Warshawsky, Cristina Boccuti.
      p. cm.
Includes bibliographical references and index.
   ISBN 0-8157-1013-5 (pbk. : alk. paper)
   1. Medicare—Congresses. 2. Long-term care of the sick—United States—
Finance—Congresses. 3. Long-term care of the sick—Government policy—United
States—Congresses. 4. Insurance, Long-term care—United States—Congresses.
I. Moon, Marilyn. II. Warshawsky, Mark. III. Title.
   RA412.3.B58 2003   2002154002
   362.1'6'0973C   dc21

9 8 7 6 5 4 3 2 1

The paper used in this publication meets minimum requirements of the American
National Standard for Information Sciences—Permanence of Paper for Printed
Library Materials: ANSI Z39.48-1992.

Typeset in Times Roman

Composition by Stephen McDougal
   Mechanicsville, Maryland

Printed by Victor Graphics
   Baltimore, Maryland

NATIONAL ACADEMY OF·SOCIAL INSURANCE

The National Academy of Social Insurance is a nonprofit, nonpartisan organization made up of the nation's leading experts on social insurance. Its mission is to promote understanding and informed policymaking on social insurance programs through research, public education, training, and the open exchange of ideas. Social insurance encompasses broad-based systems for protecting workers and their families against economic insecurity and ensuring access to health care. The Academy's work covers Social Security, Medicare, workers' compensation, unemployment insurance, public assistance, and private employee benefits.

Preface

THIS BOOK IS based on papers delivered at the fourteenth annual conference of the National Academy of Social Insurance, held January 24–25, 2002, at the National Press Club in Washington, D.C. The conference examined policies for long-term care and for chronic care and included recommendations for Medicare and other public and private programs. The Academy received financial support for this conference from the Robert Wood Johnson Foundation, the W. K. Kellogg Foundation, the John A. Hartford Foundation, and the TIAA-CREF Institute.

As with all activities organized under its auspices, the Academy takes responsibility for ensuring the independence of this book. Participants in the conference were chosen for their recognized expertise and with due consideration of the balance of disciplines appropriate to the program. The resulting papers are the views of the presenters and are not necessarily those of the officers, board, or members of the Academy.

The editors would like to thank all of the conference participants for sparking a lively discussion and debate. We also commend the Academy staff for their help in designing stimulating sessions and for facilitating the smooth running of the conference—in particular, Elizabeth Dulaney, Greg Denney, Grace Gang, Terry Nixon, Kate Robie, Cecili Thompson, and Ken Williams.

We appreciate the efforts of all those who made this book possible: the authors, for their attention to the task of turning their presentations into chapters; Krista Dowling at the Urban Institute, who assisted the editors; Pamela Larson of the Academy staff, who organized the process; Katherine Kimball, the manuscript editor for Brookings; the indexer, Robert Elwood; the proofreader, Carlotta Ribar; Janet Walker, who oversaw the project at Brookings; and the staff of the Brookings Institution Press.

Contents

1

Overview

Cristina Boccuti, Marilyn Moon,
David Blumenthal, and Mark Warshawsky

THE FOURTEENTH annual conference of the National Academy of Social Insurance, held in January 2002, took on a tough challenge: to motivate attendees to be concerned about an issue of unmet need in a time of declining government revenues and economic prosperity. The baby boomers are aging, and a considerable share of them will need long-term care, as their parents do now. The conference participants addressed ways to increase both the provision and the quality of long-term care to meet these current and absolutely predictable needs and also explored Medicare's role in smoothing the transitions between acute and long-term care.

The two-day conference, entitled Long-Term Care and Medicare Policy: Can We Improve the Continuity of Care?, grappled with these issues, considering a variety of funding options in addition to Medicare. The conference chairs, David Blumenthal, Marilyn Moon, and Mark Warshawsky, asked participants to consider the impact of acute-care policies on long-term and chronic care. Their goal was to draw attention to how the segmentation of health-care provision (by setting and by payment sources, for example) can force disruptions in patient care, creating both inefficiencies and unhelpful complexities for patients and families—often during health crises. Participants provided insight into the barriers to access and affordability between stages of disease and proposed some solutions. Even the speakers, however, often found it difficult to make linkages across the varying policy and research communities.

This volume presents papers by most of the conference participants. The material is divided into five parts, organized around the conference's panel session topics. An epilogue presents official remarks from national policymakers who were keynote speakers at the conference. The authors of these papers comprise a broad range of researchers, policy analysts, and policymakers who have had a long-standing interest in the area of long-term care. In many ways

1

the issues raised are similar to those they have expressed over the past twenty years. Little progress has been made in resolving these issues, however, although in some areas greater awareness and consensus has evolved.

First, there is a recognition that long-term care, which provides supportive services to help infirm individuals with their basic functioning, cannot and should not be thought of as fully separate from the care provided to those with chronic conditions. Both raise issues concerning acute medical care. Good chronic care can reduce long-term-care needs, and long-term care may be an essential part of treatment for those with severe chronic conditions. These areas are often separated, however, by sources of financing, by experts in each area who inadequately communicate with one another, and by attitudes regarding acute versus long-term care. Indeed, although the conference sought to bring these issues together, this proved to be a difficult task for most participants.

Second, caregiving is raised as a major theme by many of the authors, who stress the need to incorporate the wishes of the patient and his or her family or other caregivers. Third, the limitations of Medicaid in meeting the long-term-care needs of Americans are well understood. An insurance approach would not only guarantee that people would receive good care when they need it but would allow them to maintain financial security, as well.

However, the next step, consensus on how to achieve protection for persons in need of long-term care, is still beyond our grasp. The biggest divide is over whether to rely on the public or the private sector for both the resources and structure for an improved long-term-care system. Unlike the debate in the 1980s over long-term-care approaches, expectations for major public resources to help support individuals have been scaled back considerably. Proposed solutions seem to be limited to incremental approaches, even from those who believe that personal responsibility can never fully fill in the gaps.

Chronic and Long-Term Care: What Are the Needs?

Part 1 of this volume provides a description of the needs of long-term-care recipients and the methods by which they receive services. The authors also present a number of aspects of chronic and long-term care that need attention and improvement, particularly with respect to individuals' access to care and provider reimbursement. Quickly evident in this section (and throughout the book) is the range of definitions applied to the term *long-term care.*

Christine Bishop, of the Schneider Institute for Health Policy, presents her understanding of critical definitions: what is long-term care, who needs and uses it, and who supplies it. Bishop writes that an important theme in chronic and long-term care is its principal reliance on basic human intervention rather than on technology and medicine. That is, people who need long-term care are defined by their dependence on human assistance to accomplish everyday activities. Bishop notes that though rates of disability increase with age (approximately 35 percent of people age 85 and older live with a disability), about 20 percent of the disabled adult population is under the age of 65. Furthermore, recent research has shown a decline in disability rates attributable, in part, to advances in acute care.

Bishop raises a crucial point, echoed throughout the conference: the most important providers of long-term care are the patient's family and friends, but policy concerns tend to focus instead on the most expensive provider, the nursing home. Indeed, the majority of adults with long-term-care needs reside not in nursing homes but in their communities, though tracking more precisely the time and dollars expended for indirect and unpaid caregiving is difficult with the survey tools currently available.

Offering additional insight into the realities of long-term care in the United States is Robyn Stone, from the Institute on the Future of Aging Services. Stone notes that, despite the high statistical likelihood that policymakers will be touched by the issue of long-term care, either directly or indirectly, there is a strong disconnection between the public financing necessary to help defray those costs and the incentives it creates. Out-of-pocket expenses for long-term care, for example, are high—accounting for one-third of the national long-term-care bill, not including the value of unpaid work provided by family members. Furthermore, federal barriers to integrating Medicare and Medicaid impede a cohesive delivery system, except in a few exemplary cases. Private long-term-care insurance covers only a small proportion of our long-term-care expenditures. Stone asserts that this market remains largely unavailable because few individuals can afford the products.

In contrast with acute care, where medical cure is the focus, patients and their families want long-term care to focus on quality of life. Therefore, Stone suggests, adequate consumer information on nursing-home quality requires further development and commitment from the Centers for Medicare and Medicaid Services. Public information campaigns should also encourage consumers to learn more about long-term-care options before they experience health crises—a difficult charge, considering the unwillingness of many to anticipate living with a chronic, debilitating illness.

Robert Friedland, of the Center on an Aging Society, raises concerns about the quality of care that can be provided when payment for services along the continuum of illness is divided into discrete units. Comparing long-term-care coverage to a jigsaw puzzle, Friedland comments that though different incentives and eligibility criteria, when combined, make for a collection of pieces that can help, they have not yet been sorted into a coherent package of affordable long-term-care options. Family caregiving currently fills in much of the gap.

It is because of this family support that many people needing long-term care can live at home and, depending on where they live, find community-based services, turning to nursing homes only as a last resort. Friedland outlines some of the other long-term-care settings (for example, group homes and assisted-living facilities), reinforcing the observation that long-term care has a broad definition. Furthermore, options for anticipating the financial risk consist mostly of saving, moving into an insured continuing-care retirement community, and purchasing long-term-care insurance.

These options can be expensive, as acknowledged by Maribeth Bersani, from Sunrise Assisted Living. Speaking from the provider community, Bersani notes that innovations in assisted living are seen primarily in private-pay markets that serve wealthier consumers. In line with Stone's call for more consumer choice and facility accountability, Bersani stresses that in her organization active ombudsmen, representing residents, challenge their facilities to find a balance between patient freedom and patient safety.

Ingrid McDonald, from the Service Employees International Union, provides insight into the work-force crisis occurring in facilities like those Bersani represents and, even more so, in nursing homes. McDonald cautions against accepting shortsighted solutions that perpetuate the already high turnover rates in staff. McDonald states that primary considerations for increasing worker retention should address three essential aspects: wages, workload, and work environment. In light of Bishop's and Stone's characterization that patients' chronic- and long-term-care needs depend most heavily on human assistance, improving the situation of workers in the long-term-care industry is especially relevant to achieving quality care.

Paul Yakoboski, from the American Council of Life Insurers, writes that the relatively low level of participation in the long-term-care insurance market is a function of its youth, having been in existence for only fifteen years. He suggests that to increase participation, consumers need to be informed that long-term-care insurance is primarily an issue of individual retirement-income security: in 2000, the average yearly cost of staying in a nursing home was $55,000. Furthermore, in research conducted by the American Council of Life Insurers over the past year, 98 percent of insured individuals said that preparing for long-term-care expenses is an important part of their retirement planning. This interest, therefore, suggests that, as Robyn Stone also notes, consumer education is critical, especially with the aging of the baby boomers around the corner.

Although these authors approach long-term care from different points of view, on some issues they all agree. For example, all comment that work-force issues need further attention, especially considering the importance of valuing and quantifying home-care needs. Several authors also note that public financing can be inadequate in many cases and that targeted increases in reimbursement could be helpful. Most agree that the expansion of private insurance products could benefit the industry of long-term care as well as the beneficiaries of that care.

Care for the Elderly and Disabled under the American Social Contract

Although this book's title juxtaposes "Medicare" and "long-term care," Medicare does not specifically cover long-term care. Through postacute care benefits (that is, home health care and skilled-nursing-facility services), Medicare covers some of the same services needed by long-term- and chronic-care patients. This overlap, however, has never been an explicit commitment to financing long-term care. To open part 2, Theodore Marmor, a professor at Yale University, offers an explanation for why long-term care is absent from Medicare's operational and political agendas, relying primarily on historical decisions and events. Marmor posits that Medicare was designed as the first step toward universal health insurance against the costs of acute episodes of illness or injury, and thus its scope was narrow from its inception. He argues further that the role of Medicaid as a means-tested program covering room and board, as well as specific services, for low-income nursing-home residents has effectively prevented Medicare from expanding into long-term-care coverage. In this respect, Medicaid offers both social and medical benefits. However, Medicaid, by design, does not provide the social effect of income protection—a benefit that is currently available only in the private market. Moreover, Marmor asserts, there has been steadily growing support for market-based initiatives, under the premise that governments do not work.

Marmor notes an important distinction between private insurance and social insurance: whereas private insurance links the premium costs to beneficiary risk, under social insurance an individual's financing contributions are not proportional to his or her expected health-care use. Social insurance disconnects experience from premiums. In Medicare, for example, people contribute a proportion of their wages; under private insurance, members are charged a premium based on an actuary's estimation of their likely use of medical care. In this regard, Marmor argues, long-term care is an ideal candidate for social insurance, whereby people of all incomes, ethnicities, and medical conditions can contribute a small share of their incomes against the possibility of needing extremely expensive services.

In addition to the elderly, Medicare's social contract includes people with disabilities under the age of 65—a segment of the Medicare population often overlooked in popular press accounts. Among the many chronic conditions that render individuals disabled enough to qualify for Medicare is HIV/AIDS. Indeed, notes Chris Collins, of the health policy consulting company Progressive Health Partners, almost one-quarter of federal spending on health care for HIV/AIDS comes from the Medicare program. Collins presents findings from field research he conducted with June Eichner, of the National Academy of Social Insurance, investigating the role of Medicare in financing HIV/AIDS services. They observe several problems that are not unique to the disabled population but are particularly troublesome for those with HIV/AIDS (such as the twenty-nine-month waiting period and the absence of prescription drug coverage). Collins and Eichner report that the Medicare application process has been an entrance barrier to the Medicare program, as is declining physician participation. When disability can be linked to medical conditions, Medicare can play a substantial role.

Also commenting on Medicare's social contract to the elderly and those with disabilities is Michael Hash, from Health Policy Alternatives and a former deputy administrator for the Centers for Medicare and Medicaid Services. Like Marmor and Friedland, Hash attributes Medicare's failure to cover long-term care to its original design and to the establishment of Medicaid for those with low incomes, a factor in the strong institutional bias for care of the frail elderly. In response to Collins's HIV/AIDS examples, Hash notes that the Medicare-related problems faced by people with HIV/AIDS are a function of Medicare's failure to support the coordination, planning, assessment, and integration of care services. Hash suggests that more demonstration projects for "dual eligibles," those individuals who are entitled to both Medicare and Medicaid, could lend some insight into better coordination of publicly financed health care.

Coordinating care to treat diseases from the acute- to the long-term-care stages is a particular problem for people who have difficulty entering the health-care system at the acute-care stage. Shelley White-Means, of the University of Memphis, raises this concern, specifically for minorities, who have been found to underutilize acute-care services, especially physician services. Furthermore, several options that have been introduced to help people prepare for potential long-term-care needs, such as retirement communities, long-term-care insurance, and saving for long-term care, are unavailable to people with low incomes, resulting in their disproportionately high reliance on Medicaid and Medicare.

As highlighted in these summaries, the authors in part 2 raise a number of issues for the Medicare program, even if it never becomes a key player in long-term care. Coordination of acute and long-term care across payers and settings is likely to be an especially important piece of any effort to improve the delivery and quality of care for those with chronic conditions.

Prospects for Long-Term-Care Policymaking at State and Federal Levels

Political environments affect the acceptance and design of health-care reform. Almost everyone interested in long-term care, whether from the perspective of researcher, provider, insurer, or consumer advocate, is keenly aware that any changes to the status quo of long-term care will involve government intervention. National and state policymakers play critical roles in initiating improvements in the provision and financing of long-term care.

Beginning the discussion, in part 3, on the prospects for long-term-care policymaking at state and federal levels, Judith Feder, the dean of policy studies at Georgetown University, offers some political comparisons across recent long-term-care reform proposals. She notes that though President Bill Clinton's Health Security Act included two large-scale initiatives (both in financing and benefits) to increase access to home care and long-term care, these proposals received little or no political attention. In contrast, the 1995 budget debate on transforming Medicaid from an individual entitlement program to a state block-grant program aroused considerable political discussion—ultimately allowing the threat of capped federal funds to become a more engaging and impassioned issue than the improvement of beneficiary access to long-term care.

So how can a more offensive strategy be initiated to improve long-term-care services and financing? Feder suggests that policymakers need to recognize long-term care as the unpredictable, unmanageable event that it is—naturally requiring insurance to spread the risk. She argues that trust in government will also play a major role, if public sources are called upon to finance the increased need for long-term care. Feder cites work from the U.S. General Accounting Office highlighting the government's role in oversight, particularly in regard to the quality of nursing-home care. Feder thus anticipates a continuing and important role for government.

In some cases, however, government needs to get out of the way, notes Ruth Katz (speaking on behalf of John Hoff), from the Office of the Assistant

Secretary for Planning and Evaluation in the Department of Health and Human Services. States can often be most effective and creative when the federal government is involved as a silent partner. Katz commends the work of many states in offering innovative long-term-care solutions, particularly those participating in Cash and Counseling Demonstrations designed to give consumers more choice and control over their care. Results from this project include high consumer satisfaction rates. According to Katz, President George W. Bush is committed to loosening federal controls that present obstacles to long-term-care service delivery, as can be seen in the Olmstead Executive Order, calling for agencies to find ways to eliminate barriers to the receipt of home- and community-based services.

Federal involvement and initiatives, also, can directly improve access to and quality of long-term care. Katz cites, for example, the Administration on Aging's Caregiver Support Program, designed to assist family and friends who provide care to people at home. Katz sees a federal role in raising awareness for long-term-care planning, including long-term-care insurance options. Moreover, states Katz, consumer information disseminated by the U.S. Department of Health and Human Services can help to dispel misperceptions that Medicare covers long-term care in nursing homes. Commenting on the conference theme of continuity of care, Katz writes that with respect to patient assessment instruments, primary- and acute-health-care systems do not generate good record-keeping or communication with one another. The Office of Planning and Evaluation has a long-range goal to streamline health-care records to span acute-, primary-, and long-term-care settings so that providers can access patient information at any time along the continuum of care.

Joshua Wiener, of the Urban Institute, reminds readers that even with this federal involvement, states generally hold the reins in long-term-care reform. Simply put, states have a stronger fiscal stake and are more involved in the day-to-day operations in long-term care. States have a greater opportunity for reform because they can be more flexible than the federal government. Wiener's decades of research reveal that though some states are innovative and spend both money and time on home- and community-based services, others have instituted no significant improvements in this area. As a result, eligibility for services varies between states—a fact that raises concerns about horizontal equity and warrants federal involvement.

Is Medicare the right player to call on for increased federal involvement in long-term care? Wiener suggests that Medicare may be too bureaucratic to be able to account for local and individual needs and therefore is not the best vehicle for reforming the long-term-care system. He recommends that we turn instead to models of state and federal partnerships, such as the State Children's Health Insurance Program (SCHIP)—a politically popular and rather successful initiative. With its high federal match and state flexibility, SCHIP contains many of the long-term-care features of Clinton's health reform proposal mentioned earlier by Feder.

David Durenberger, a former senator from Minnesota and the current director of Citizens for Long-Term Care, explains why long-term-care policy is not on legislative agendas. Besides being overshadowed by overriding national security concerns, he suggests, long-term care is a problem that the public does not want to address because it is thought to be too close to issues concerning the end of life. If advocates could attach long-term-care issues to current legislative agenda items such as financial security, Durenberger posits, they might be more successful in attracting policymakers' attention. Essentially, he proposes a strategy that would use current economic stimulus proposals as a "wedge" for introducing long-term-care reform. He suggests further that long-term care could even be connected to national security because personal financial security hinges on the asset protection aspect of long-term care.

John Rother, of AARP, also comments on the need to politically ignite the issue of long-term care. Rother agrees with Feder and Wiener that the federal agenda does not place enough importance on long-term-care reform. He attributes the lack of activism to people's fear of the topic and lack of education on their potential need for long-term care. Rother reports that AARP is on the verge of launching a multiyear effort to increase its members' understanding of the range of options, from independent living through long-term care to end of life.

Long-term care is not only off the federal government's "to do" list; it is not high on the major media's topic list, either. Joanne Silberner, of National Public Radio, describes some of the limitations on reporting on long-term-care issues. This topic does not fit well into the category of "news" because it has not experienced major legislative changes in the last decade. Narrative stories are occasionally run, but without sexy headlines their appeal to editors is limited. Silberner says that there is hope, however, because editors, most of whom are baby boomers, are likely to gravitate toward stories that affect them personally. This is good news for the issue at hand, because many of those editors are beginning to confront their parents' needs for long-term care.

As elsewhere in this volume, the authors presented in part 3 make a number of suggestions to improve long-term care and its coordination across service settings. What distinguishes these suggestions is the extent to which the recommendations are made in light of political realities. Many propose strategies for attracting political attention to the issue of long-term care, acknowledging that even the best reform design is worthless if policymakers ignore the issue.

Building on Experience: What Have We Learned about Meeting Needs for Chronic and Long-Term Care?

Aware that the audience would eventually hear about many problems with our nation's long-term care, the conference chairs organized a panel that presented models of success. Part 4 of this book provides some discussions on innovative systems that have worked in providing long-term care. The authors make suggestions for reform based primarily on specific lessons they have learned in their respective fields of expertise.

Improvement in the quality of care is often listed as an important goal for long-term-care reform but is rarely outlined in specific steps and strategies. However, the first author presented in part 4, Catherine Hawes, a professor in the Department of Health Policy and Management at Texas A&M and the director of the Southwest Rural Health Research Center, does point to concrete ways to improve the quality of long-term care, backed by her own research findings. First, she states that government regulation can improve quality, noting the overall positive effect of the Omnibus Budget Reconciliation Act of 1987. Hawes praises the federal role in quality improvement, observing that it is more collaborative with the providers than state governments. She notes that the Minimum Data Set created by the Centers for Medicare and Medicaid Services and other resident assessment tools can, if used correctly, help providers (as well as watchdog agencies) monitor the performance of their facilities over time.

Hawes also notes from her other recent research that nursing-home residents in states with the least regulation have had higher rates of hospitalization and faster rates of cognitive, functional, and physical decline than those in states with greater regulation. She suggests, therefore, that increased regulation and improved quality of care can lower costs. Hawes introduces another success story in long-term care—the Wellspring model—in which staff teamwork and empowerment have contributed tremendously to a reduction in turnover rates without an increase in costs.

Bruce Fireman, a biostatistician, relays his experience with disease management programs for chronic conditions at Kaiser Permanente, a nonprofit managed-care organization. The diseases currently being addressed at Kaiser Permanente are coronary heart disease, heart failure, diabetes, asthma, complex chronic conditions (most relevant to the frail elderly), chronic pain, and hypertension. Some key components of these programs include databases for use in identifying appropriate participants, drug protocols, and even motivational interviewing to encourage life-style changes. He finds that enrollees in disease management programs have fared better on quality indicators than eligible nonenrollees, even after adjustments for risk and selection bias. Patient satisfaction is also high for members in these chronic-care management programs.

Despite the theory that higher-quality care could lead to reduced hospitalizations, Fireman notes that utilization trends for Kaiser Permanente's disease management patients do not differ significantly from those in the general adult Kaiser member population. Thus, he concludes, there has been little change in total costs for treating members in these programs beyond what is attributable to trends in the general Kaiser population and to inflation in the costs of medical care. Based on these results, Fireman suggests that the promises of disease management be articulated in terms of cost effectiveness rather than cost savings.

Focusing on chronic care for Medicare beneficiaries, Marty Lynch, who recently completed work with colleagues at the Institute for Health and Aging at the University of California at San Francisco, presents and discusses several initiatives in service provision. His project examined chronic-disease-care and long-term-care models, all of which attempt to bring together acute- and long-term-care services—with varied success. Lynch reports that the Program of All-Inclusive Care for the Elderly (PACE) has been the most successful at this mission, while the social health maintenance organization programs, in contrast, have been disappointing. Lynch cites the EverCare model as the best example of a residential program whose staff works in multidisciplinary teams. Lynch and his colleagues have found promising models for disease management with examples in Kaiser Permanente and Group Health, among others. Lynch states that although comorbidities were not well addressed, patient satisfaction and reduced emergency room and hospital admissions have resulted from several disease management models.

One missing element in these models, Lynch writes, is that there is no crossover between the models for disease management and residential care. As a result, long-term-care programs are not incorporating disease management principles into their service delivery. Lynch also finds little in the way of disease management for Medicare beneficiaries in fee-for-service provision. He suggests that Medicare find a method of case management for high-risk beneficiaries in fee-for-service provision that could carry them into long-term care, if needed. Similarly, he recommends integration of home- and community-based care to help avoid cost shifting and improve care for consumers.

Several authors in part 4 praise the PACE programs—and in particular, On Lok, the pioneer PACE—for making strides in the integration of acute and long-term care as well as the merging of the Medicare and Medicaid "silos." Jennie Chin Hansen, the executive director of On Lok, offers comments on these accomplishments in light of the program's slower-than-expected growth. The Program of All-Inclusive Care for the Elderly has been successful in providing a continuum of care to its patients by employing an integrated and interdisciplinary team of health-care providers. The customized nature of the care that PACE enrollees receive owing to their frailty, however, has contributed to the slow growth of the program. Clients in PACE, who average eight medical comorbid conditions, bowel incontinence, and functional dependencies, require personalized care, which presents growth challenges, because economies of scale allow only a small gain in a staff-intensive, care-intensive environment. Hansen also attributes PACE's slow growth to start-up challenges; the initial capital needed for PACE programs is large and relatively uncertain, given the risk-adjusted payment system. Consequently, few providers are willing to make the investment.

Bruce Vladeck, currently at Mount Sinai Medical Center, responds to these authors' recommendations with an observation made during his tenure as the administrator of the Health Care Financing Administration: the implementation of new programs, including long-term-care reform, will not save Medicare any money, despite frequent assurances to the contrary. Vladeck also reminds readers that Medicare bears much of the financial burden of increasing life expectancies. Medicare's ability to take on more long-term-care liability, therefore, poses a distinct financial challenge in addition to those presented by the complicated nature of long-term care. He writes that long-term-care advocates and analysts who complain about the slow progress of long-term-care reform should recognize how difficult it is to serve the complex needs of frail, disproportionately poor individuals with limited family resources.

Visions for the Future: How Might We Meet Tomorrow's Needs for Chronic and Long-Term Care?

The aging of the baby-boom generation and decreasing funds for long-term care warrant swift solutions on ways to meet the impending demand. Part 5 presents authors' recommendations and analyses on meeting the future need for long-term care. Although he was unable to attend the conference, John Cutler, from the U.S. Office of Personnel Management (OPM), presents in this volume a discussion of the OPM's recent offer of long-term-care insurance to federal employees and qualified relatives (including parents). The design and outcomes of the federally managed long-term-care insurance program will have significant bearing on the shape of tomorrow's long-term-care insurance market.

Cutler expects that, like the health and life insurance programs the OPM administers, the Federal Long Term Care Insurance Program will become the largest employer-sponsored long-term-care insurance program in the nation. The Federal Long Term Care Insurance Program product is fully portable, so employees can maintain their long-term-care insurance after leaving government employment. To increase applications further, the private insurers with which the OPM has contracted are organizing education campaigns to raise federal employees' awareness of the importance of long-term-care insurance and the incapacity of Medicare, Medicaid, and their health insurance to cover much of long-term care, should they need it.

According to Cutler, the employer-sponsored product offered by the Federal Long Term Care Insurance Program will be able to stay contemporary to compete with the policies offered by other employers. The OPM plans to keep abreast of changes in how long-term-care services are provided and to make appropriate changes in policy. By statute, there will be no government contribution to the premium, as is the case with individually purchased long-term-care insurance. This lack of subsidy distinguishes the product from other federal employee benefits such as health insurance. Also in contrast to the health benefit program, applicants to the federal long-term-care insurance program may be denied coverage by the contracted insurers because underwriting is allowed.

Mark Warshawsky, currently with the U.S. Department of the Treasury, further explores the private sector. Based on collaborative academic research, Warshawsky proposes a new insurance product to address the problems facing the individual long-term-care insurance market. He suggests the creation of an integrated annuity product that packages long-term-care insurance with an immediate life annuity, thereby keeping good and bad risk in the same pool and increasing the interest and the number of applicants. Consistent with the private market approach, his proposal emphasizes individual responsibility and personal choice and minimizes the contribution from public programs.

Empirical work on this proposal recently appeared in the *Journal of Risk and Insurance*, in which Warshawsky and his colleagues, Christopher Murtaugh and Brenda Spillman, estimate that the population of people attracted to this integrated product would be larger than the population who would purchase each element separately. Based on this result, therefore, an integrated product could achieve greater risk protection in the long-term-care insurance market because it could make policies more attractive, thus making participation available to more people. Warshawsky notes that public policy issues on the implementation of this integrated insurance product require further research and review. For example, taxation questions, the level of Medicaid involvement, and regulatory authority are all concerns that can be addressed during or after its implementation.

In thinking about future reform, Mark Merlis, a seasoned health policy analyst, presents an international comparison of long-term-care systems. Merlis cites a wide array of public approaches that exist outside the United States. Comparing shares of public spending on long-term care, he notes that the United States falls somewhere between the middle and the bottom, depending on details of accounting methodology. However, the United States differs from the other countries in requiring impoverishment before any public contributions are made. One alternative occurs in Belgium and the Netherlands, where sliding-scale coinsurance is a part of the payment mix from the outset.

Merlis also finds that elderly people in the United States who need publicly subsidized housing are more likely to reside in nursing homes than are their counterparts in other selected OECD countries, where housing options such as old-age homes and hostels are more common than in the United States. This difference may suggest that we examine whether public funding toward less intensive—and potentially less expensive—housing would be a more efficient use of our resources. Public policies on informal caregiving may also play a role in rates of nursing-home use. Merlis writes that whereas some countries pay family caregivers directly for providing long-term-care services, other countries hold siblings financially liable for services rendered to those receiving long-term care.

Discussion of long-term-care reform often has the potential for ignoring and possibly removing the personal nature of long-term care, as found in some of Deborah Stone's research. Stone, a professor at the Rockefeller Center at Dartmouth College, challenges several assumptions of policymaking in her chapter. She argues that rationalizing care—assigning discrete cost and time units to each and every service—does not result in more care for less money. Successful long-term care relies on building good relationships between caregivers and the patients who need them, but as Stone points out, time for this component is not reimbursable.

Stone notes that among many elements of home care, building patient-provider rapport is hard to price, and thus third-party insurers are unaware of what really happens during home-health-care visits. Stone also points out that the least well paid members of provider organizations—the certified nursing assistants—are probably the most valuable to the patient and his or her family. Stone suggests that in creating a future with more caring long-term-care communities, we also reevaluate the assumption of rampant overutilization in long-term care and find a way to reward caregivers for the compassion and warmheartedness they exhibit in treating frail, elderly patients.

Similarly focused on the personal aspects of long-term care, Monsignor Charles Fahey, of the Milbank Memorial Fund, also defines, with personal stories rather than statistics, the present and future populations in need of long-term care. He highlights recent progress for two groups of people with handicapping conditions—those born with assistance needs and those who acquire a disability at a relatively young age. These people will need services for all or most of their lives. Monsignor Fahey notes that the *Olmstead* decision, the Willowbrook Consent Decree, and vibrant advocacy have helped move society to foster inclusiveness for persons with disabilities. Lessons here may be applied to the frail elderly in the sense that institutional care should be avoided unless absolutely necessary, because people usually want to stay in their homes and in their communities.

Richard Bringewatt, from the National Chronic Care Consortium, defines chronic illness as exhibiting five characteristics: it is multidimensional, interdependent, disabling, ongoing, and personal. He stresses that long-term-care policy should be careful to address each of these components and avoid the financial incentives that encourage health-care providers to avoid the sickest patients in some cases and overhospitalize in others. Bringewatt writes that current long-term-care policy focuses on diagnosis and disease rather than functional needs, which are more personal. In keeping with the conference theme of continuity of care, Bringewatt also suggests standardizing provider participation requirements across care settings because chronic disease often progresses through several settings.

Agreeing with Bringewatt that long-term care is less about health care than about personal life-style maintenance, William Scanlon, the director of Health Care Issues at the U.S. General Accounting Office, provides perspectives from his experience as a policy analyst for Congress and as a former long-term-care researcher and economist. Scanlon suggests that a lack of consensus on the objectives for long-term-care policy has been an obstacle to progress in reforming long-term care. He asserts that there is little agreement on what benefits should be guaranteed and what financial protections should be afforded.

Scanlon applauds Warshawsky's proposal to improve the long-term-care insurance marketplace. He cautions, however, that even if the private long-term-care insurance market begins to grow rapidly, the public sector will retain a significant role in financing long-term care with respect to policy affordability and private costs, especially for policyholders whose needs become extremely expensive. Commenting on Mark Merlis's presentation comparing long-term-care systems abroad, Scanlon notes that it is difficult to evaluate the differences between systems when we know little about the consequences of their varying levels of public and private subsidization.

Part 5 reflects the closing panel of the two-day conference. In line with all the previous authors and discussants, the authors of these chapters concur that reform is necessary to ensure that those requiring long-term care in the future are able to access the services they need. Although the private market for long-term-care insurance is growing slowly, its pace is likely to increase as more people learn about the product and as the federal employee program gets under way. For some people, however, policymakers and providers will need to find ways to improve financing as well as service delivery and productivity. Social insurance, thus, can play an instrumental role in finding solutions to the current and future inadequacies of long-term care in the United States. Indeed, social insurance, perhaps in partnership with the private sector, is quintessentially suited for equitably insuring against the risk of a devastatingly expensive, generally arbitrary event that requires long-term-care services.

Conference Summary

Overall, the conference saw points of consensus and points upon which differences of opinion were expressed. All conference participants agreed that long-term care could be an insurable event and that insurance is a better mechanism for providing financing for most of the population than the current Medicaid welfare program. All participants also agreed that the existence of insurance would lead to improvements in the economic status of workers in this sector, just as the spread of health insurance led to the improvement of the economic status of workers in the acute-health-care sector. Finally, there was agreement that more research needs to be done and statistics need to be collected to better test policy ideas and ascertain trends.

Differences of opinion were expressed about the relative roles of the private and public sectors in providing insurance for long-term-care needs. Private long-term-care insurance is a growing and rapidly changing product (albeit on a small base), but further developments and innovations are possible. Some ideas have been proposed here to expand the role of social insurance programs, as well. Clearly, a careful balance and integration will need to be achieved, as they have in the retirement income area, where private savings, employer-sponsored pension plans, and Social Security coexist.

Finally, finding ways to strengthen the intersection between long-term care and chronic care was a steep challenge for most participants. Indeed, many stated that the Program of All-Inclusive Care for the Elderly remains the only successful paradigm for bridging the two types of care. As a program limited to the very frail, however, PACE is either unavailable to or the wrong model of care for many people with chronic- or long-term-care needs. Currently, we have no consensus on how to integrate and bridge the medical care afforded in the chronic-care sector with the assistance provided in long-term care. Further efforts are greatly needed to develop flexible approaches that allow coordination and interchange between services provided in these two sectors of care.

PART ONE

Chronic and Long-Term Care:
What Are the Needs?

2

Long-Term-Care Needs of Elders and Persons with Disability

Christine Bishop

THE INTERFACE BETWEEN long-term- and acute-care services is complex and problematic. These two types of care address different needs, are supplied by overlapping providers, and are financed from different sources, yet they serve many of the same individuals. This conference volume represents a welcome in-depth consideration of long-term-care policy issues with an added challenge: that we consider also how acute-care policy might help or hinder policy goals for long-term care. This chapter draws on available statistics and recent research findings of others to provide definitions and background useful for considering these issues. It is organized around a number of questions: What is long-term care? Who needs and uses long-term care? Who supplies long-term care? What are critical aspects of the interface between acute and long-term care?

Long-term care and acute or chronic care have different objectives: the focus of long-term care on assistance that compensates for functional disabilities has wide-ranging implications for the provision and use of this care. Moreover, the demarcation between household-based and provider-based surveys hinders knowledge about the people who need and use long-term care and leaves some of them uncounted. The most important providers of long-term care are the family and friends of people with long-term-care needs, but policy concerns tend to focus instead on the most expensive provider, the nursing home, which appears to be in transition, with a changing role in the long-term-care system. In the American system, care for acute health conditions is likely to be covered by private insurance and Medicare, whereas long-term care is generally paid for out-of-pocket or by Medicaid. There are opportunities for efficiency in the overlap of populations who need both these types of care, as persons with long-term-care needs also have greater-than-average needs for acute care. Furthermore, broader access to advances in acute care may be able to reduce future demand for long-term care by reducing the likelihood of disability in the future.[1]

What Is Long-Term Care?

Long-term-care services support daily living activities of people with functional limitations. Functional limitations often result from insults to health—acute and chronic illness or injury—but in its strictest definition, long-term care does not deal with the illness that may have caused these problems. Rather, it compensates for the chronic functional disability that the illness or injury has caused.

This makes long-term care quite different conceptually from health care for acute and chronic conditions. The objective of the former service is assistance with everyday living functions rather than amelioration or cure of disease. Just as patients value health services because they improve health outcomes, individuals with disabilities value long-term-care services because they allow them to carry out what are called activities of daily living (ADLs) and instrumental activities of daily living (IADLs). The former are the ordinary activities, including eating, dressing, and getting to the toilet, that we tend to take for granted.[2] The latter are everyday activities that are instrumental for independent living, including managing money, using the telephone, preparing meals, and doing laundry, and enable people to live independently.[3] Although some functional difficulties can be addressed with equipment of various kinds, assistance from another person is usually the key input in providing long-term care. This is critical to many of the dilemmas we face in our long-term-care system.

---

1. For further background, the reader is also referred to current reviews of long-term-care issues and policy, including Robert B. Friedland and Laura Summer, *Demography Is Not Destiny* (www.agingsociety.org/demograp.htm [November 5, 2002]); Stone (2000); W. Spector and others, "The Characteristics of Long-Term Care Users" (www.ahcpr.gov/research/ltcusers/index.html#tables [November 5, 2002]); National Center for Health Statistics (2001); and Cutler (2001).

2. The five main ADLs are transferring (getting into and out of a bed or chair), bathing, dressing, eating, and toileting. A sixth is getting around inside.

3. The IADLs are preparing meals, shopping for groceries, doing the laundry, using the telephone, performing light housework, taking medications, managing finances, and getting around outside.

Who Needs and Uses Long-Term Care?

An accurate estimate of the number and characteristics of people who need and use long-term care is surprisingly hard to come by. Household surveys do not cover the institutions and group quarters in which a substantial number of persons with long-term-care needs live.[4] This makes it hard to obtain comparable information on needs and services for the entire population of persons with disabilities. Surveys of providers report information on people receiving care in certain institutions, but the surveys are restricted by institutional definitions. This narrow institution-by-institution view may once have provided adequate continuous estimates of long-term-care populations and their needs. In the past decade, however, institutions like nursing homes have been shifting their roles and the populations they serve, and new sites for long-term care are emerging in the marketplace. The services and needs of residents in assisted-living facilities, congregate housing, and foster care are not well captured by either institution-focused or household-focused surveys.

. The National Long-Term Care Survey is an exception, in that it provides information on the disability needs of people regardless of where they live or how they receive care; but it is limited to persons aged 65 and older, and many people who need assistance with activities of daily living are not elderly. Although the decennial census does not focus on disabilities and care, it does survey the entire population regardless of residence. Data on disability and type of residence, however, are not yet available from the 2000 census. Despite these data limitations, in 1995 the Office of the Assistant Secretary for Planning and Evaluation (ASPE) in the U.S. Department of Health and Human Services pieced together data for 1990 from various sources into a composite picture to make several points that almost certainly are still true today. The ASPE analysis shows clearly that the population in need of long-term care includes many younger people as well as elders. Two-fifths of the adults needing personal assistance because of disabilities are under the age of 65. Moreover, most adults with long-term care needs do not reside in institutions but rather live in their communities. This holds true for both the elderly and younger adults (figure 2-1).

4. See, for example, analysis of the Survey of Income and Program Participation reported in Centers for Disease Control and Prevention (2001b) and reports based on the National Health Interview Survey follow-back disability supplement for 1994–95 (NHIS-D)—for example, Kennedy (2001) and S. Larson and others, "Functional Limitations of Adults in the U.S. Noninstitutionalized Population: NHIS-D Analysis" (rtc.umn.edu/nhis/databrief5/MRDDDBOct01.pdf [November 5, 2002]).

Figure 2-1. *Adult Population Needing Long-Term Care, by Age and Care Setting, 1990 (estimate)*

Thousands of persons

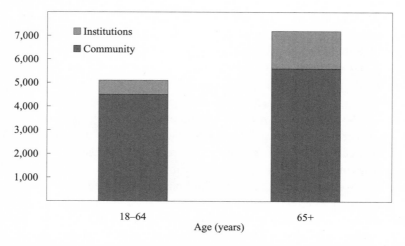

Age (years)

Source: Author's calculations based on data from Michelle Adler, "Population Estimates of Disability and Long-Term Care," table 2 (http://aspe.hhs.gov/daltcp/reports/rn11.htm [November 5, 2002]).

Although many persons in need of long-term care are not elderly, the prevalence of need for personal assistance experienced by persons living in the community increases with age (figure 2-2). The prevalence of need for assistance is quite low, under 5 percent, from age 15 to 55 and then begins to rise. The group aged 80 and older has substantial risk of needing assistance, although this is not inevitable for elders who survive into these later years. According to these estimates, even among persons aged 80 and older, only 35 percent have need for assistance with activities of daily living.

Who Supplies Long-Term Care?

Long-term care is provided by residential providers, formally organized community-based providers, independent workers, and family and friends. Residential providers include nursing homes, assisted-living facilities, group homes, and foster care. Home-health-care and home-care agencies provide long-term care to people with disabilities in their own homes, and persons needing long-term care who reside in their communities also use out-of-home day services, like adult day care and adult day health care. Paid home helpers

Figure 2-2.   *Need for Personal Assistance among Community-Resident Adults, by Age, 1997*

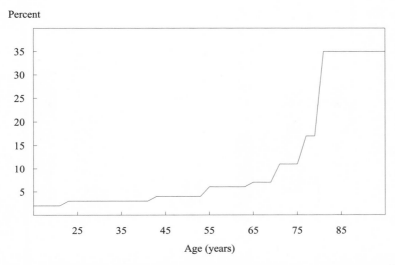

Percent

Source: Author's calculations based on data from Jack McNeil, "Americans with Disabilities: 1997," U.S. Department of Commerce, Bureau of the Census, Household Economic Studies, P70–73, February 2001 (www.census.gove/prod/2001pubs/p70-73.pdf [November 5, 2002]).

also play a role, but it is not possible to estimate how much of domestic workers' labor is disability support—in part, because of gaps in formal employment records for these workers. The most important providers of long-term care, however, are family members and friends of those in need of personal assistance.

Most community-resident elders with disability needs rely on assistance from family members. Figure 2-3, based on data collected by the 1994 National Long-Term Care Survey, presents estimates of the use of various combinations of paid and informal care by elders with substantial needs for long-term assistance. It is important to note the sheer numbers of these elders who are managing to remain in the community. However, it is quite unusual for elders to remain in their community residences with paid assistance only, especially as their needs increase. (The figure shows elders in nursing homes and other institutions as relying on paid care only. It should be noted, however, that some of them also have ongoing assistance from family and friends who come in to help.) Most people with ADL and IADL needs who live in the community rely on unpaid help only or on a combination of paid and unpaid assistance.

Figure 2-3.   *Use of Paid and Informal Long-Term Care by Community-Resident Elderly, by Level of Disability, 1994*

Thousands of persons (estimate)

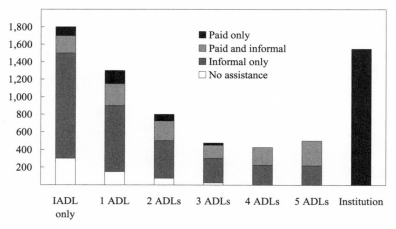

Source: Author's calculations based on data from Liu, Manton, and Aragon (2000, tables 1 and 2).

Note: In this figure and others in this chapter, IADL = instrumental activities of daily living; ADL = activities of daily living.

The National Long-Term Care Survey data also indicate that average weekly hours of care provided to elders living in the community rise as long-term care needs increase (figure 2-4). Elders with greater needs receive more care from family members and other informal sources. Multiplying the numbers of elders at various levels of need (figure 2-3) by the average weekly hours of care by level of need yields a rough estimate of the total hours of care supplied in a typical year for elders with disabilities—a whopping 5.3 billion hours of care in the year. Four-fifths of this is unpaid care provided by family and friends (figure 2-5).[5] This unpaid care represents a tremendous resource provided to elders in our society.

An old rule of thumb states that for every elder in a nursing home, two others with similar needs are living in the community. Reliable, objective information on the level of independence in activities of daily living for elders in nursing homes is difficult to obtain because staff do so much for institutional residents, just by the nature of the institutional setting. For example, nursing-home

5. Calculated by the author from Liu, Manton, and Aragon (2000). This result, though very large, is still substantially smaller than estimates computed using surveys of caregivers rather than individuals with disabilities—for example, Arno, Levine, and Memmott (1999).

Figure 2-4. *Average Weekly Hours of Formal and Informal Long-Term Care of Community-Resident Elderly, by Level of Disability, 1994*

Care hours per person

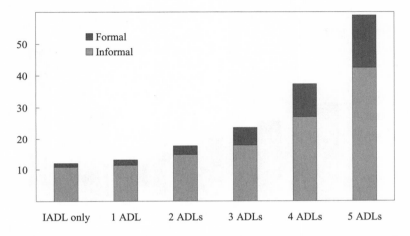

Source: Author's calculations based on data from Liu, Manton, and Aragon (2000, tables 3, 5, and 6).

residents rarely bathe without assistance, even when they are able to do so. We can, however, get a rough idea of the level of disability of elders in nursing-home and community-care settings by combining data from the National Long-Term Care and National Nursing Home Surveys (figure 2-6). This indeed suggests that at least as many elders with high levels of need are being cared for in the community as in nursing homes.

The national health accounts can track dollars going to certain types of providers—nursing homes, home-health-care providers, and durable medical equipment suppliers—but these expenditures include postacute, rehabilitative, and some chronic health care as well as assistance for disability-related needs. The national health accounts do not track paid assistance that is not specifically health related, such as the long-term-care-related aspects of congregate housing or expenditures for a housekeeper who prepares meals and helps with medicines for older persons who cannot do these activities on their own. The total expenditure for the providers that can be tracked was $143 billion in 2000—13 percent of all personal health expenditures.[6] Long-term-care expen-

6. Centers for Medicare and Medicaid Services, "National Health Expenditures by Type of Service and Source of Funds: Calendar Years 1960–2000" (www.hcfa.gov/ stats/nhe-oact [January 15, 2002]).

Figure 2-5.   *Yearly Hours of Paid and Informal Long-Term Care of Community-Resident Elderly, by Level of Disability, 1994 (estimate)*

Millions of care hours

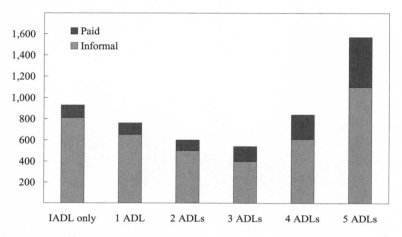

Source: Author's calculations based on data from Liu, Manton, and Aragon (2000).

ditures loom especially large in Medicaid budgets, making up 35 percent of the total in 2000. Nursing-home care is the largest expense, accounting for 8.2 percent of total expenditures on personal health and 20 percent of total Medicaid spending. Care for younger persons with disabilities also captures a large share of Medicaid spending, with 5 percent of total spending going for institutional care for persons with developmental disabilities and 9 percent for community-based care, much of which is expended to meet the needs of those with developmental disabilities.

The most expensive provider of long-term care, the nursing home, appears to be in the midst of a transition.[7] Data from the National Nursing Home Survey suggest a continuing decline in the rate of use of nursing-home care for the oldest elderly (figure 2-7). Nursing-home occupancy rates have been falling, as have the number of private-pay residents.

The decline in occupancy rates comes as a surprise both to those who have been bracing for the increased long-term-care needs of an aging population and to the industry itself. In the search for explanations, some have pointed to the downward trends in age-adjusted rates of disability, but these declines are small and cannot account for the decline in use. Instead, the downward trend in

7. See Bishop (1999).

Figure 2-6. *Care Settings of the Elderly, by Level of Disability (estimate)*

Percent of those aged 65 and over

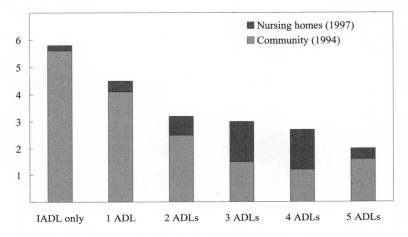

Source: Author's calculations based on data from Liu, Manton, and Aragon (2000) and Celia Gabrel, "Summary: Characteristics of Elderly Nursing Home Current Residents and Discharges: Data from the 1997 National Nursing Home Survey," National Center for Health Statistics, *Advance Data from Vital and Health Statistics*, no. 312 (April 25, 200) (www.cdc.gov/nchs/data/ad/ad312.pdf [November 5, 2002]).

nursing-home use appears to be a function of shifting configurations of the services offered by various long-term-care providers. First, the nursing home itself is changing: nursing homes responded to changes in Medicare policy during the 1990s by orienting themselves more toward postacute care, including rehabilitative therapies, and thus somewhat less toward traditional long-term care. This is reflected in their case mix: the disability and health needs of their residents have been increasing over time. Second, in response to rising incomes and some public policy changes, other care settings are emerging in the marketplace. Elders with disabilities who can pay for their own care are now likely to seek home-delivered services or care in assisted-living facilities rather than nursing-home care. The emerging residential settings are not counted with the traditional nursing-home institutions, although some look very much like the nursing homes of twenty and thirty years ago.

One important fact shaping long-term care today is that, for the most part, it is not covered by insurance. Nursing-home care, in particular, can result in catastrophic expense for individuals and families. Twenty-seven percent of this care is paid for out-of-pocket, compared with 16 percent of other health services. Public funding covers only a defined portion of residential long-term

Figure 2-7.   *Use of Nursing Homes by Age, 1985, 1995, and 1999*

Residents per 1,000 population by age

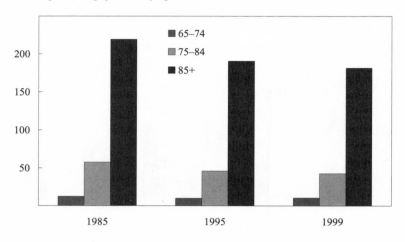

Source: Author's calculations based on data from National Center for Health Statistics, "National Nursing Home Survey," 2002 (www.cdc.gov/nchs/about/major/nnhsd/nnhsd.htm [November 5, 2002]), and Bishop (1999).

care: Medicaid pays for about half the nursing-home bill, but only for persons who are poor or who have become poor through their spending on nursing-home care. Medicaid does not generally cover the emerging residential settings. Medicare and private insurance appear on the list of nursing-home payers, but they cover postacute care for patients with high rehabilitative and acute care needs rather than residents with disability-related needs for assistance. The population covered by private long-term-care insurance is growing in response to improving insurance products and increasing awareness of the catastrophic financial risks of future long-term-care needs, but coverage is still not widespread. The distribution of payment sources suggests that markets and public policy place a higher priority on access to life-saving services for persons with acute health problems than on access to supportive services for elders with disabilities.

Interface between Acute-Care and Long-Term-Care Services

Despite the distinctions that separate long-term-care and acute-care services, there are benefits to considering them together. First, people with disability needs tend to have greater needs for health services as well, so that

Figure 2-8.   *Average Medicare Expenses per Beneficiary by Level of Disability and Care Setting, 1991 to 1994*

Dollars per person

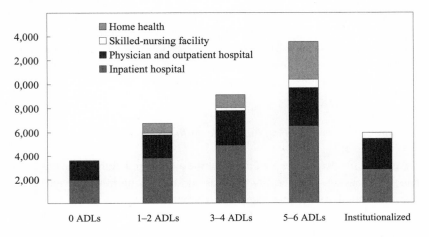

Source: Author's calculations based on data from Riley (2000, table 6).

there may be gains from managing these services together. Second, it appears that acute-care services, as well as life-style changes, are driving recent downward trends in disability. These trends will not be maintained without continuing improvements in access to advances in health care.

Persons with Disabilities Use More Acute-Care Services

Estimates of the average expenses by level of disability indicate that for community-resident Medicare beneficiaries, acute-care expenditures increase as disability increases (figure 2-8).[8] Average Medicare expenditures are significantly greater for beneficiaries with functional disability than for the estimated 63 percent of beneficiaries with no ADL needs. The use of inpatient hospital care, physicians' services and outpatient hospital care, skilled-nursing-facility (SNF) care, and home health care increase as disability needs increase for community-resident beneficiaries. However, average inpatient

8. This point is also made by Feder and Lambrew (1996), who do not distinguish institutional residents.

hospital and postacute (SNF and home health) expenditures for nursing-home residents at all levels of disability are lower than those for any of the categories of community-resident beneficiaries with ADL needs. Care-management programs have been developed to capitalize on possible efficiencies in the joint provision of acute- and long-term-care services. These include the social health maintenance organization, EverCare, and the federal Program of All-Inclusive Care for the Elderly (PACE).[9] The coordination of acute- and long-term-care services is an important future direction for the interface between long-term- and acute-care provision and financing.

Acute-Care Services Affect Future Needs for Long-Term Care

Age-specific death rates are falling for the older population, and average life span is increasing. Past fertility patterns and improving mortality mean that increasing numbers of Americans are achieving the age ranges at which the risk of disability has been highest. But many of the diseases and conditions that cause death also cause disability. As these diseases are mitigated, it is plausible that age-specific disability rates might fall in concert with mortality rates, and they have been doing just that: the decline in age-adjusted disability rates is estimated at .56 percent per year (figure 2-9).[10] In the words of a recent report, these declines appear to be "consistent, widespread, and robust."[11] This has important implications for society's plans for long-term-care provision and financing. If disability rates continue to fall, long-term-care needs will be less overwhelming than was previously expected.

It is important that the composition and possible sources of these declines in disability be understood so that they can be perpetuated. A substantial portion of the decline in the rates of disability as measured by dependence in ADLs and IADLs has occurred in the rates of dependence in the IADLs (see figure 2-9). The IADL dependencies often reflect impairments in cognitive function. Population surveys consistently show improvement in the age-adjusted preva-

9. On the social health maintenance organization, see Leutz and others (1991), Leutz (1992), Kane and others (1997), and Boult and Pacala (1999). On EverCare, see Kane and Huck (2000); on the Program of All-Inclusive Care for the Elderly, see Eng and others (1997), Lee and others (1998), Rudolf and Lubitz (1999), and Master and Eng (2001).

10. Manton and Gu (2001, p. 6356). Aspects of the debate on this issue are succinctly summarized in Freedman and Martin (2000).

11. Schoeni, Freedman, and Wallace (2001, p. S206); see also Freedman, Aykan, and Martin (2001), Manton and Gu (2001), and Cutler (2001).

Figure 2-9. *Disability Rates of Elders, by Level of Disability, Selected Years, 1982–99*

Percent

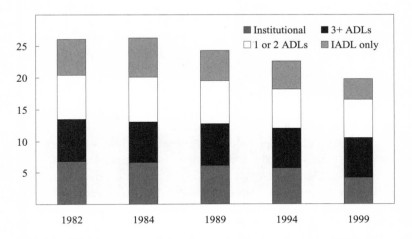

Source: Author's calculations based on data from Manton and Gu (2001, table 1).

lence of cognitive functional deficits at rates that are faster than the declines in physical disabilities.[12] Falling rates of cognitive impairment are associated with the increasing educational attainment of the elderly population, a trend that is expected to continue into the future.[13] A portion of the reported decline in IADL needs may also derive from positive changes in consumer services markets: people report fewer difficulties with such activities as grocery shopping, preparing meals, managing money, doing laundry, and using the telephone when delivery services, computer banking, and improved household appliances and communication devices are widely available to assist consumers in general.[14] Although these market changes might be masking changes in underlying functional disability, they also suggest the promising prospect that markets can respond to the needs and demands of aging consumers.

12. Freedman (2001); Manton and Gu (2001).
13. Freedman and Martin (1999).
14. Unpublished work by Brenda Spillman and colleagues (Spillman 2001) has highlighted this aspect of the decline in reported disability. Elders may respond that they are not experiencing difficulty with shopping, for example, because of the availability of grocery delivery services, whereas they would have experienced difficulty without such services. The decline in disability, and its impact on the ability of elders to remain independent in the community, is no less real because of this market effect.

Medical advances and receipt of medical care are believed to be responsible for a substantial portion of the recent declines in functional disability and have the potential to support a continuing downward trend in disability rates.[15] Childhood exposure to infectious disease has been strongly linked with disability in old age, so that the improved past treatment of current aging cohorts should continue to reduce functional disability.[16] Improvements in the treatment of heart disease and stroke have reduced both mortality and morbidity resulting from these cardiovascular conditions.[17] Better early detection of certain cancers has lowered cancer-related disability as well as cancer mortality.[18] Elders who can move through their arthritis thanks to more effective symptom control can delay mobility impairments.[19]

It is intriguing that the prevalence of chronic conditions is increasing (see figure 2-10) simultaneously with declines in the prevalence of disability associated with chronic diseases and conditions.[20] It is possible that chronic conditions are being more widely diagnosed and treated, thereby reducing their ability to cause functional limitations.[21] Prescription drugs in development directed toward the problems of elders have the potential to contribute further to these trends (figure 2-11).

Life-style changes, most notably the decline in smoking, have also led to decreased mortality and morbidity and are likely to support the trend of falling disability rates into the future.[22] Working against disability declines are persistent and worsening rates of poor diet, insufficient exercise, and excessive alcohol consumption.[23] Rather than making health-care services less relevant, however, these life-style effects illustrate how the acute-care sector can sup-

15. Boult and others (1996); Freedman and Martin (2000); Blackwell, Hayward, and Crimmins (2001).

16. Costa (2000); Blackwell, Hayward, and Crimmins (2001).

17. Centers for Disease Control and Prevention (1999); Cutler, McClellan, and Newhouse (1999); Cutler and others (1998); Zelinski and others (1998); Freedman and Martin (2000).

18. Wilmoth (2000).

19. Reynolds, Crimmins, and Saito (1998); National Academy for an Aging Society, "Arthritis" (www. georgetown.edu/research/ihcrp/agingsociety/profiles/arthritis.pdf [November 5, 2002]).

20. Federal Interagency Forum on Aging Statistics, "Older Americans 2000: Key Indicators of Well-Being," indicator 14 (www.agingstats.gov [March 21, 2002]).

21. Freedman and Martin (2000).

22. Centers for Disease Control and Prevention (2001a).

23. Hubert and Fries (1994); Serdula and others (1996); Vita and others (1998); Stuck and others (1999).

Figure 2-10.   *Selected Chronic Conditions among Persons Aged 80 and Older, by Sex, 1984 and 1995*[a]

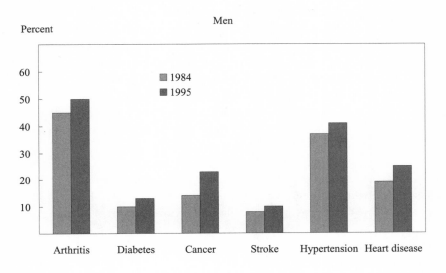

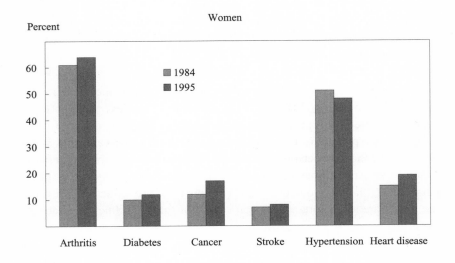

Source: Federal Interagency Forum on Aging Statistics, "Older Americans 2000: Key Indicators of Well-Being" (www.agingstats.gov [March 21, 2002]).
    a. 1984 percentages are age adjusted to the 1995 population. The reference population is the civilian noninstitutional population.

Figure 2-11. *Medical Conditions of the Elderly Targeted by New Drug Therapies*

Number of drugs in development

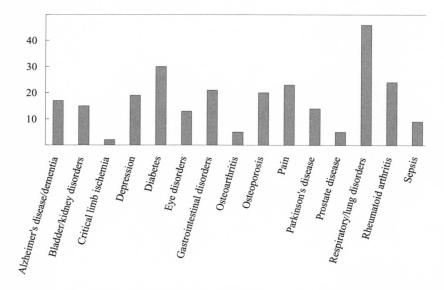

Source: Pharmaceutical Research and Manufacturers of America, "New Medicines in Development for Older Americans," 2002 (www.phrma.org/mediaroom/press/releases/28.06.2002.443.cfm [October 29, 2002]).

port the personal changes that are critically important to the reduction of morbidity and disability. Medical research continues to uncover links between health and life-style choices. Although health counseling to convey this information to patients is not always a part of standard health care, consumers often receive the most personalized and powerful information about the effects of tobacco, alcohol, fitness, and obesity from their own physicians or other personal health-care providers. Improvements in life-style factors, whatever the cause, are an important potential source of future declines in disability rates.

Summing Up

Long-term care is personal assistance to compensate for disabilities. This is what makes it so expensive now and will make it more so in the future. The technological changes that are affecting so many aspects of modern production and modern life are unlikely to have much impact on a service that consists of hours of hands-on one-to-one care. Public policy concerned with meeting long-term-care needs must focus on the staffing of institutions and agencies, the training of workers, wages and benefits adequate to attract and retain those workers, and family caregivers. The dearth of opportunity for efficiency gains darkens the prospect of an aging baby-boom population, with fewer adult children to serve as caregivers and little possibility for technological "fixes."

There are glimmers of hope on the horizon, however—most notably, in financing innovations that could better prepare for and spread future personal risks of high need but also for the reduction of need itself. Researchers are uncovering a strong causal link between health services that prevent, defer, treat, and mitigate acute and chronic diseases and conditions and the disability caused by disease and injury. With our financing system skewed as it is toward acute care, and severely underfinanced for provision of assistance with every-day tasks, there is an irony here: a key part of long-term-care policy must be to make current medical treatment—particularly the prescription drugs that can defer and ameliorate chronic disease—available to more people, old and young, who could benefit from these medical advances.

References

Arno, P. S., C. Levine, and M. M. Memmott. 1999. "The Economic Value of Informal Caregiving." *Health Affairs* 18 (2): 182–88.

Bishop, C. E. 1999. "Where Are the Missing Elders? The Decline in Nursing Home Utilization, 1985–1995." *Health Affairs* 18 (4): 146–55.

Blackwell, D. L., M. D. Hayward, and E. M. Crimmins. 2001. "Does Childhood Health Affect Chronic Morbidity in Later Life?" *Social Science and Medicine* 52 (8): 1269–84.

Boult, C., and J. T. Pacala. 1999. "Integrating Healthcare for Older Populations." *American Journal of Managed Care* 5 (1): 45–52.

Boult, C., and others. 1996. "Decreasing Disability in the Twenty-First Century: The Future Effects of Controlling Six Fatal and Nonfatal Conditions." *American Journal of Public Health* 86 (10): 1388–93.

Centers for Disease Control and Prevention. 1999. "Achievements in Public Health, 1900–1999: Decline in Deaths from Heart Disease and Stroke, United States, 1900–1999." *Morbidity and Mortality Weekly Report* 48 (30): 649–56.

———. 2001a. "Cigarette Smoking among Adults: United States, 1999." *Morbidity and Mortality Weekly Report* 50 (40): 869–73.

———. 2001b. "Prevalence of Disabilities and Associated Health Conditions among Adults: United States, 1999." *Morbidity and Mortality Weekly Report* 50 (7): 120–25.

Costa, D. L. 2000. "Understanding the Twentieth-Century Decline in Chronic Conditions among Older Men." *Demography* 37 (1): 53–72.

Cutler, D. M. 2001. "Declining Disability among the Elderly." *Health Affairs* 20 (6): 11–27.

Cutler, David M., Mark McClellan, and Joseph Newhouse. 1999. "The Costs and Benefits of Intensive Treatment for Cardiovascular Disease." In *Measuring the Prices of Medical Treatments,* edited by J. E. Triplett, 34–71. Brookings.

Cutler, D. M., and others. 1998. "Are Medical Prices Declining? Evidence from Heart Attack Treatments." *Quarterly Journal of Economics* 113 (4): 991–1024.

Eng, C., and others. 1997. "Program of All-Inclusive Care for the Elderly (PACE): An Innovative Model of Integrated Geriatric Care and Financing." *Journal of the American Geriatric Society* 45 (2): 223–32.

Feder, Judith, and Jeanne Lambrew. 1996. "Why Medicare Matters to People Who Need Long-Term Care." *Health Care Financing Review* 18 (2): 99–112.

Freedman, V. A. 2001. "Recent and Future Changes in Cognitive Functioning among Older Americans." Paper presented at Private Long-Term Care Insurance Conference, August.

Freedman, V. A., H. Aykan, and L. G. Martin. 2001. "Aggregate Changes in Severe Cognitive Impairment among Older Americans, 1993 and 1998." *Journals of Gerontology Series B: Psychological Sciences and Social Sciences* 56 (2): S100–11.

Freedman, V. A., and L. G. Martin. 1999. "The Role of Education in Explaining and Forecasting Trends in Functional Limitations among Older Americans." *Demography* 36 (4): 461–73.

———. 2000. "Contribution of Chronic Conditions to Aggregate Changes in Old-Age Functioning." *American Journal of Public Health* 90 (11): 1755–60.

Hubert, H. B., and J. F. Fries. 1994. "Predictors of Physical Disability after Age Fifty: Six-Year Longitudinal Study in a Runners Club and a University Population." *Annals of Epidemiology* 4 (4): 285–94.

Kane, R. L., and S. Huck. 2000. "The Implementation of the EverCare Demonstration Project." *Journal of the American Geriatric Society* 48 (2): 218–23.

Kane, R. L., and others. 1997. "S/HMOs, the Second Generation: Building on the Experience of the First Social Health Maintenance Organization Demonstrations." *Journal of the American Geriatric Society* 45 (1): 101–07.

Kennedy, J. 2001. "Unmet and Undermet Need for Activities of Daily Living and Instrumental Activities of Daily Living Assistance among Adults with Disabilities: Estimates from the 1994 and 1995 Disability Follow-Back Surveys." *Medical Care* 39 (12): 1305–12.

Lee, W., and others. 1998. "PACE: A Model for Integrated Care of Frail Older Patients: Program of All-Inclusive Care for the Elderly." *Geriatrics* 53 (6): 62, 65–66, 69, 73.

Leutz, W. 1992. "Recognizing the Achievements of the Social Health Maintenance Organization (SHMO) Demonstration Sites." *Journal of Aging and Social Policy* 4 (3–4): 9–12.

Leutz, W. N., and others. 1991. "Adding Long-Term Care to Medicare: The Social HMO Experience." *Journal of Aging and Social Policy* 3 (4): 69–87.

Liu, K., K. G. Manton, and C. Aragon. 2000. "Changes in Home Care Use by Disabled Elderly Persons: 1982–1994." *Journals of Gerontology Series B: Psychological Sciences and Social Sciences* 55 (4): S245–53.

Manton, K. G., and X. Gu. 2001. "Changes in the Prevalence of Chronic Disability in the United States Black and Nonblack Population above Age 65 from 1982 to 1999." *Proceedings of the National Academy of Sciences* 98 (11): 6354–59.

Master, R. J., and C. Eng. 2001. "Integrating Acute and Long-Term Care for High-Cost Populations." *Health Affairs* 20 (6): 161–72.

National Center for Health Statistics. 2001. *Trends in Health and Aging.* Hyattsville, Md.

Reynolds, S. L., E. L. Crimmins, and Y. Saito. 1998. "Cohort Differences in Disability and Disease Presence." *Gerontologist* 38 (5): 578–90.

Riley, G. F. 2000. "Risk Adjustment for Health Plans Disproportionately Enrolling Frail Medicare Beneficiaries." *Health Care Financing Review* 21(3): 135–48.

Rudolph, N. V., and J. Lubitz. 1999. "Capitated Payment Approaches for Medicaid-Financed Long-Term Care Services." *Health Care Finance Review* 21 (1): 51–64.

Schoeni, R. F., V. A. Freedman, and R. B. Wallace. 2001. "Persistent, Consistent, Widespread, and Robust? Another Look at Recent Trends in Old-Age Disability." *Journals of Gerontology Series B: Psychological Sciences and Social Sciences* 56 (4): S206–18.

Serdula, M. K., and others. 1996. "The Association between Fruit and Vegetable Intake and Chronic Disease Risk Factors." *Epidemiology* 7 (2): 161–65.

Spillman, Brenda. 2001. "Declines in Elderly Disability Rates: What Really Has Changed?" Paper presented at Private Long-Term Care Conference. LTC Insurance Educational Foundation, Miami, August 19–22, 2001.

Stone, Robyn. 2000. *Long-Term Care for the Elderly with Disabilities: Current Policy, Emerging Trends, and Implications for the Twenty-First Century.* New York: Milbank Memorial Fund.

Stuck, A. E., and others. 1999. "Risk Factors for Functional Status Decline in Community-Living Elderly People: A Systematic Literature Review." *Social Science of Medicine* 48 (4): 445–69.

Vita, A. J., and others. 1998. "Aging, Health Risks, and Cumulative Disability." *New England Journal of Medicine* 338 (15): 1035–41.

Wilmoth, J. R. 2000. "Demography of Longevity: Past, Present, and Future Trends." *Experimental Gerontology* 35 (9–10): 1111–29.

Zelinski, E. M., and others. 1998. "Do Medical Conditions Affect Cognition in Older Adults?" *Health Psychology* 17 (6): 504–12.

3

Reality of Caring for the Long-Term-Care Population

Robyn Stone

AS A LONG-STANDING member of the National Academy of Social Insurance, I am pleased to write about the realities of long-term care. I have been pressing the academy specifically to address the issues of long-term care for a number of years. I was excited, therefore, to see it prominently featured as the major subject of the 2002 annual meeting.

Long-term care rests on four cornerstones: financing, delivery, work force, and consumer information and education. I believe there are six realities that are key for policymakers, researchers, providers, and the general public to understand. These realities reflect the unique nature of the long-term-care policies and programs present in the United States and the barriers and opportunities we face in developing a more coherent system of services and support.

The Four Cornerstones of Long-Term Care

In previous work I have referred to the "triple knot" of long-term care— financing, delivery, and work force. I have since revised my vision to a rectangle. The framework has been expanded to include what may be the most important part of the foundation: consumer information. As our programs offer more options to individuals and their families, consumers must both make initial decisions and navigate increasingly complicated financing and delivery systems.

Financing Long-Term Care

As Christine Bishop noted in chapter 2, Medicaid is the largest payer of the long-term-care bill, its share representing approximately 40 percent of all expenditures. This program continues to have an institutional bias, although over the past decade states have made a significant investment in home- and community-based services. Medicare is also a payer, although it does not cover services considered to be traditional long-term care (for example, personal-care and nonmedical home-care services and long stays in nursing homes). Medicare covers postacute stays in skilled-nursing facilities and home health care for individuals who are homebound and need skilled nursing. During the early 1990s, Medicare expenditures on home health care grew exponentially, owing in large part to an increase in the volume of home visits by health aides. Provisions in the Balanced Budget Act of 1997 substantially cut this benefit, in an effort to return the program to its postacute-care roots.

Out-of-pocket payments made by individuals and their families represent one-third of the national long-term-care bill. Private long-term-care insurance is responsible for only a small proportion of the expenditures (between 5 and 10 percent, depending on how insurance is defined). The individual insurance product, which is expensive unless purchased at a relatively young age, continues to dominate the market. Group products, which have the advantage of creating larger risk pools and providing more affordable options, have not been aggressively developed. Given the instability of the employer-based health insurance market, however, it is unlikely that most employees would contribute to the development of a market for long-term-care insurance. Consumer ignorance about the risk of needing long-term care has also deterred the evolution of this market. Consequently, the future of group long-term-care insurance is uncertain. The new federal long-term-care insurance option recently offered for the first time to all federal employees and retirees will be one interesting experiment to watch over the next decade. Although it is not employer subsidized, the program has the potential to create the largest-ever insurance pool and to test the viability of long-term-care insurance for a substantial population of working-age individuals.

Delivery of Long-Term Care

Over the past decade, policymakers, researchers, and innovative providers have expounded on the virtues of a long-term-care continuum that would provide an array of service and setting options for individuals as their needs and preferences change over time. I prefer the concept "repertoire of services and settings" because "continuum" has a linear connotation that usually suggests a downward trajectory. In fact, people with long-term-care needs have a more dynamic trajectory, with the potential for improvement as well as deterioration and the interweaving of episodes of acute as well as chronic care.

A responsive long-term-care delivery system, therefore, must be flexible enough to meet these changing demands and should provide mechanisms for coordinating services across settings and providers.

Long-term care implies services that run the gamut from assistance with personal hygiene and other activities of daily living to medication management and skilled nursing. For many individuals, however, assistive technology ranging from canes and walkers to emergency alert systems and home modifications from grab bars in bathrooms to universal design throughout the home may be just as important as hands-on care, and perhaps more so.

Despite attempts by some policymakers, providers, and researchers to create a cohesive delivery system, the United States has witnessed surprisingly little innovation over the past three decades. Long-term care remains fragmented, and there are few examples of effective and sustained coordination of services and supports. A number of states (Arizona, Wisconsin, and Oregon, for example) have pooled long-term-care dollars and have had varying success in developing managed long-term-care systems. Federal barriers to full integration of Medicare and Medicaid, however, have made it difficult for states or providers to effectively coordinate services across the spectrum from acute to primary to long-term care.

The Program of All-Inclusive Care for the Elderly (PACE) represents a model of successful financial as well as service delivery integration, but its providers serve only the most disabled, nursing-home-certifiable older adults, and enrollment in their programs tends to be small. EverCare is one model that has attempted to integrate primary care with long-term-care services for nursing-home residents. After years of operation in a number of sites, this approach is still being evaluated, and the extent of success remains to be seen. Several home-care providers (for example, the Visiting Nurses Service of New York) are experimenting with coordination of primary- and long-term-care services for their target populations, but the results of these initiatives are not yet available.

The buzzword of long-term care over the past two decades has been assisted living, a catchall phrase that denotes a congregate living arrangement with supportive services to meet the needs of older adults and younger people with disabilities. The evidence to date, however, suggests that this model has been developed primarily as a product for relatively wealthy individuals to purchase in the private market. Several researchers have argued that this model is frequently expensive and is relatively short on assistance, particularly for people with cognitive impairment. A few states (Oregon and Washington) have aggressively used the Medicaid waiver authority to create assisted-living programs for low-income individuals and have successfully substituted this model for more costly nursing-home care without jeopardizing the residents' quality of care or life. These are the rare exceptions, however, and we have a long way to go before affordable housing with services becomes a part of the long-term-care repertoire.

The newest trend in long-term-care policy development is consumer-directed care. This concept encompasses a diversity of options ranging from giving people a say in the development and implementation of their care plans to actually providing them cash in lieu of a service package. The majority of states include some type of consumer direction in their home- and community-based-care programs, and Arkansas, Florida, and New Jersey are participating in the Cash and Counseling Demonstration, a rigorous experiment supported by the U.S. Department of Health and Human Services and the Robert Wood Johnson Foundation. Although preliminary findings indicate that some older adults as well as younger people prefer to have cash and manage their own resources and care, this approach is not appropriate for everyone. Furthermore, policymakers will have to decide how to balance consumer autonomy and choice with the safety and protection of clients.

The Long-Term-Care Work Force

The third cornerstone of long-term care, the work force, is perhaps the most important and most neglected of the policy concerns. Even if we were to solve our financing dilemma tomorrow, a coherent long-term-care delivery system would not emerge without a prepared, stable, qualified work force. The long-term-care work force in the United States is presently in crisis, and without significant policy intervention, the problem is certain to escalate in the future.

There are not enough clinicians across the professional spectrum (physicians, nurses, therapists, social workers) trained in geriatrics and qualified to deliver long-term care, to coordinate services, and to manage care across the repertoire of providers and settings. There are not enough trained administrators and managers able to provide leadership in this labor-intensive field. There are not enough direct-care workers—certified nursing assistants, home-care aides, personal-care attendants—who provide most of the daily hands-on care needed by people with disabilities. It is not enough simply to recruit "warm bodies." We need to prepare and sustain a quality paraprofessional work force to support the long-term-care delivery system. Finally, informal caregivers are ill prepared to meet the clinical, physical, and emotional needs of their disabled or infirm family members, especially in light of these three professional shortages.

The development of a high-quality, stable long-term-care work force will come about only through an integrated policy approach that goes beyond long-term-care reimbursement, regulation, and program design. It will require an assessment of the interactions among education, labor, welfare, and immigration policies and of the strategies that encourage these sectors to work together at both the federal and state levels to create positive incentives for work-force development. It will also require that providers of long-term care create work environments that attract new workers at all levels to the field and, more important, encourage them to remain in the field.

Consumer Information and Education

Consumer choice in health and long-term care has become the mantra of many policymakers in Washington and across the states. This is a vacuous promise, however, in the absence of the knowledge with which to make informed choices. Consequently, consumer education is the fourth cornerstone of long-term-care policy. Polls and media reports indicate that despite attempts by the Centers for Medicare and Medicaid Services and state agencies to increase awareness about long-term care, public understanding of this issue, including its definition and range, the lack of public benefits, service and setting options, and financing strategies, is severely limited. Most long-term-care decisions, furthermore, are made at a time of crisis, with little or no prior planning.

A comprehensive consumer information and education strategy must include initiatives that address the status of current programs and benefits and the gaps in those programs, how to make service, setting, and provider choices, navigate the system, assess and monitor the quality of services provided, and resolve conflicts. Judicious consumer choices do not just happen. Similarly, consumer education and dissemination of information are not "free goods." Policymakers must recognize that resources are required to educate consumers, including an investment in aging- and disability-friendly materials and mechanisms for reaching various target populations. Consumer report cards, such as those being tested through the Centers for Medicare and Medicaid Services' recent nursing-home quality initiative, will be at best benign and at worst confusing and misleading without adequate education about how to interpret and use the information.

The Realities of Long-Term Care

Six key issues reflect the reality of long-term care in the United States. First, the long-term-care experience is essentially universal. From a statistical and anecdotal perspective, everyone is touched by long-term care, either directly or indirectly, sometime during the life course. Despite the universality of the experience, a strong disconnection between the personal experience and policymaking levels has impeded our ability to develop a coherent long-term-care policy in this country. Although many factors influence this paradox, I believe that a pervasive ageism in our society, coupled with the view of long-term care as a death sentence and an overwhelming fear about the financial and emotional burdens it imposes, has created significant inertia around this issue.

The second reality is that the family is, and will continue to be, the major provider of long-term care. The statistics highlighted by Christine Bishop substantiate the stories of millions of caregivers—primarily women—who provide hours of unpaid care to family members with long-term-care needs. Policy discussions have shifted over time from a major concern about replacing family caregiving with formal, publicly subsidized services to a focus on how services can complement and support the informal care system.

The third reality is that services and housing are coequal partners in long-term care. Where and how one lives is as important to the quality of care and the quality of life as the services and supports that are provided. Yet most of our policy debates in long-term care focus on the service side of the equation. Although the housing dimension is clearly a part of the nursing-home bill (45 percent of Medicaid expenditures cover room and board), most policymakers do not explicitly recognize the importance of housing policy in the development of a cohesive long-term-care strategy.

The fourth reality is that both the quality of care and the quality of life are key concerns in long-term care. Unlike the medical model of acute care, which focuses primarily on curing or delaying the manifestations of disease, long-term care is primarily focused on enhancing the functional independence of individuals for as long as possible. Consequently, quality of life becomes at least as important as quality of care. As the United States moves forward with its obsession with the development of quality-of-care measures, it must be borne in mind that indicators of quality of life may be better barometers of success.

The fifth reality of long-term care is that financing is, and will likely remain, a mix of public and private mechanisms. As Bishop has noted, Medicaid and, to a lesser extent, Medicare are major public payers in long-term care, but one-third of expenditures for long-term care are out-of-pocket—and that figure excludes the volume of unpaid labor as well as the opportunity costs associated with informal caregiving.

The sixth reality is related to the previous issue. The system of financing and delivering long-term care is, and probably will remain, quite fragmented. The various pots of federal, state, and local dollars that finance long-term care in this country have created silos of services and care settings that make it difficult to develop a client- and family-centered system. This is a dilemma both for the individuals and families who are trying to access services and supports and for the providers who are trying to delivery quality care.

The Uncertain Crystal Ball

I have spent my career in long-term-care policy and research, and I find reviewing the activities of the past three decades and facing the realities at the dawn of the twenty-first century to be a disturbing exercise. Our system suffers from the lack of a coherent policy for financing long-term care, a fragmented and uncoordinated delivery system, an ill-prepared and sorely inadequate professional and paraprofessional work force, and an uninformed citizenry.

There is room for optimism, however, because the graying of the baby-boom generation will place significant pressure on our society to address the four cornerstones of long-term care. My crystal ball suggests that we will continue to pursue incremental solutions to the financing of long-term care with increased flexibility in how public dollars are spent for long-term-care options. Given our country's fondness for using the tax code to help "deserving" individuals, we will quite likely see tax breaks offered for the purchase of insurance and tax credits for receipt of long-term care and caregiving. We are unlikely to see the adoption of a social insurance approach to the financing of long-term care such as those in effect in Austria, the Netherlands, Germany, and Japan.

We will continue to experiment with new delivery models that attempt to better integrate services across settings and providers. The nursing home as we know it today will become a dinosaur, as new residential care and service models replace the mini-hospital design created in the 1960s. We will have to figure out how to deal with the transition period, as antiquated institutions make way for new homelike environments. Policymakers will eventually recognize the importance of housing policy in their struggle to develop long-term-care options for modest- and middle-income older adults as well as individuals with low incomes.

The current work-force situation looks grim, but it can only get better as demand forces us to address the supply issue. Development of the work force across the entire spectrum will become a major public policy issue, and we will see investments at the federal and state levels as well as in the private sector to encourage new leadership in the clinical and managerial areas. The future of the frontline work force is less certain, although it is clear that long-term care cannot be delivered without these low-paid workers. I am hopeful that the demographic imperative, coupled with a shift in the image of long-term care, adoption of a livable wage for caregivers, and improved work environments for workers, will help us to develop and sustain a high-quality, committed long-term-care work force. Our public policies and private sector initiatives must focus on retention because sustaining a prepared work force is, in the long run, more cost-effective than continual recruitment. We will also need to explore strategies for developing new pools of labor, including older women who may be interested in caregiving careers, former welfare recipients, and new immigrant populations.

The rhetoric around consumer choice in long-term care will continue in the future. Unless we invest resources in mechanisms for educating consumers, however, public ignorance and misinformation will remain the norm. We need to better understand the knowledge gaps and how to transmit information to various groups of consumers, including people with limited health literacy. We also need to strengthen the infrastructure of information intermediaries at the state and local levels (for example, insurance counseling programs, area agencies on aging, and local chapters of AARP, the Older Women's League, and the Alzheimer's Association). Ultimately, policymakers must assess whether an "informed consumer" is a viable concept in long-term care.

Ensuring Quality and Accountability

Stakeholders in the long-term-care arena are all demanding quality. Given the difficulties in defining and measuring this concept, we do not really know what strategies to date have been most effective in ensuring quality. Policymakers and researchers must take a hard look at the relative value of the approaches currently being pursued: regulation, litigation, ombudsman programs, voluntary accreditation, quality-assurance activities (for example, the new role for the Centers for Medicare and Medicaid Services' Quality Improvement Organizations), and internal quality improvement. What are we getting for our investments? What are the trade-offs, and could we create a better allocation of resources? The ultimate test of success should be the development of a system that works for consumers and their families and that strikes the right balance between the choice, autonomy, and quality of life it affords and the safety, protection, and quality of care it delivers.

4

Planning for and Financing Long-Term Care

Robert B. Friedland

IN SIGNING THE Social Security Act into law, President Franklin Roosevelt observed that the industrial changes of the late eighteenth and early nineteenth centuries had increased the economic insecurity of life in the United States. The law, he noted, would "give some measure of protection to the average citizen and to his family against the loss of a job and against poverty-ridden old age." The addition of Medicare and Medicaid to the Social Security cornerstone thirty years later, President Lyndon Johnson noted, insured citizens against "the ravages of illness" in old age. Because of the provisions in the Social Security Act and the private insurance that evolved to fill in gaps or build upon this protection, more and more financial risks have become pooled. The financial risks and the consequences of failure to plan for long-term care continue to grow, however, and remain a serious threat to most families.

Long-Term Care: The Invisible Issue

The public policy discussions surrounding Social Security and Medicare did not include long-term care. In part, the risks and consequences of needing this kind of assistance were less apparent in 1935 and 1965. People of all ages are now surviving acute episodes and accidents that were likely in the past to have led to death. Advances in science and the applications of biomedical research have changed the way we live and die. The longer we live, the more likely it is that we will require hands-on assistance from others for substantial

I am grateful for the support provided by the Andrus Foundation, the Century Foundation, and the Robert Wood Johnson Foundation for research on the financing of long-term care. Views expressed here are entirely those of the author.

periods of time. Based on current trends in mortality and morbidity, many more of us will need long-term care.[1]

In the absence of sustained public policy attention, long-term care has evolved at the edges of the health-care system. In many ways long-term care is defined by what it is *not* rather than what it *is*. It is not acute care. Nor is it rehabilitative care. Yet people who need acute care sometimes also need long-term-care services. Certainly those who need long-term care also need health care. Benign neglect of long-term care has enabled a health-care system to develop with fuzzy boundaries between the care covered by health insurance and health plans, on the one hand, and long-term care, on the other.

For state governments, the period of neglect changed as soon as nursing-home expenditures became substantial portions of Medicaid budgets. Deliberate policy efforts were then undertaken to find ways to reduce the rate of growth in nursing-home expenditures. Until recently, this meant limiting the construction of new nursing homes and caps on reimbursement for nursing-home residence. Only in the past decade have there been efforts among some states to expand access to home- and community-based care and personal care. These efforts, however, are undertaken primarily in the name of reducing nursing-home expenditures, not to improve the quality of life.

The Long-Term-Care Puzzle

Long-term care is like a commingling of the pieces of different jigsaw puzzles in one pile. Any piece picked from the pile is as likely as not to belong to a different puzzle from the previous piece. Different goals and objectives and different criteria for eligibility make for a collection of pieces that might be individually helpful but just do not fit together. Creating a cohesive picture is difficult, if not impossible.

A confusing array of fragmented and disjointed services and sources of assistance is not limited to long-term care; it exists to varying degrees throughout the health-care system. Relative to health care, however, long-term care is far less organized. In health care, much of the care is provided or overseen by

1. Over the past two decades, disability rates among older people have declined (Manton and Gu 2001; Cutler 2001). Disability rates increase with age, however, and so for any individual each additional year of life results in a slightly greater chance of becoming disabled. Furthermore, disability rates among people under the age of 65 have been increasing, and many of these younger people will survive to older ages (Kaye and others 1996). In the future, many more people will reach the age of 85, and thus even if disability rates among the elderly continue to decline, there are likely to be at least as many people needing long-term care in the future.

physicians. Physicians help families sort out what to do and where to go in the health-care system. No one profession, particularly none with medicine's stature, is accountable for long-term care.

Moreover, unlike health care, long-term care includes few third-party payers. This, of course, makes the family financially responsible for its decisions. However, it has also hampered the development of the delivery of long-term care. With the important exception of each state's Medicaid program, there is far less attention to the delivery of care itself. Even Medicaid, in accordance with its mission, is the payer of last resort and is not structured to devote tremendous resources to the health-services research necessary to define optimal care arrangements.

The dearth of reliable and consistent information from a professional source puts the onus on individuals in need of long-term-care services. Decisions are often made at a time of crisis. These circumstances probably contribute to inefficiencies and ineffective efforts. States are certainly aware of the difficulty in navigating the long-term-care system and to varying degrees have taken steps to make it easier, as well as to make the system more effective.[2]

Despite these efforts, however, no one is happy with the current set of arrangements. Families struggle mightily to sort out their options and implement a care plan. Those with few resources and no immediate family are at the greatest risk of reaching a crisis without the support they need. Policymakers, concerned about what is already being spent, are fearful of spending even more. This has resulted in a series of incremental efforts at the state level as they await federal action and the promise of a private insurance market.

Among the public, the single most-often identified source of long-term care is the nursing home. In 1996, there were 16,700 certified nursing facilities with a total of 1.8 million beds—near double the number of beds in hospitals (almost 1.0 million beds). Nonetheless, people feel less positive about nursing homes than about any other provider of health care. Forty-five percent of respondents in a recent survey (and 49 percent of respondents with firsthand experience with nursing homes) felt that people deteriorate after placement in a nursing home.[3] Only 12 percent said they would prefer a nursing home if they became unable to take care of themselves at home. In sharp (but probably unrealistic) contrast, 78 percent said that if their health were to deteriorate to this point, they would prefer to be in an assisted-living facility.

---

2. Coleman (1996); Coleman, Kassner, and Pack (1996); Kane, Kane, and Ladd (1998).

3. NewsHour and Kaiser Foundation (2001).

Asked how they might feel if they had been moved into a nursing home, 47 percent that they would not like it but would probably come to accept it, and 43 percent said they would find it totally unacceptable. Nursing homes are structured to provid   who need the most assistance. Nursing h   ere and is covered by   een encouraged, in part,

Despite the dread   nse of disappointment,   erm care has not yet be   kers may have fears that   ures, not the least of whi   their families.[4] Perhaps   same time. Perhaps it is   who cannot imagine be   aps it is a sense of shar   n the worry or need for   long-term care is am   ancial consequences are

The Ways and Means of Financing Long-Term Care

Among the different sources and sites of long-term care, care in an institution represents the largest monthly expense, ranging from $3,000 to $6,000 a month. It is virtually impossible to purchase the key components of round-the-clock care provided in a nursing facility for much less. Care purchased outside of an institution, however, can be purchased in smaller increments. A nurse may be hired through an agency for $20 to $40 an hour, and someone working independently may charge half as much. Similarly, the services of a personal attendant or direct-care worker might cost $12 to $15 an hour through an agency or about half that amount in the "underground" market. Long-term care might be needed for only three or four months, or it might be required for ten or more years, with varying amounts of assistance needed, ranging from a few hours a week to nearly twenty-four hours a day.

4. Families provide as much care as they can and in many cases, among primary caregivers, more than they should. In many ways the level of effort today is greater than that in the past, despite the fact that public resources covering long-term care are greater than they have ever been.

Fortunately, not everyone needs round-the-clock care. Unfortunately, those who need assistance have difficult choices to make. How much care is needed, and when? Is it the right type of assistance? Is the facility safe? What about getting to the doctor? What about avoiding isolation? Is it affordable? Although care purchased in smaller increments can, in theory, be tailored to the needs of the person receiving assistance and his or her family, in practice that goal is hard to achieve. People who need care may need it at sporadic times during the day and night. Eating, sleeping, and using the bathroom are not activities that can be easily scheduled from 9:00 a.m. to 5:00 p.m. Monday through Friday.

Medicare finances care in nursing homes (skilled-nursing facilities only) and through home-health-care agencies (though not all home care is provided through a Medicare-certified home-care agency), but though some of this care is help with the activities of daily living, most is either postacute and rehabilitative care or ancillary care associated with the need for postacute or rehabilitative care. Other public financing of long-term care includes programs funded through the Older Americans Act and programs for veterans as well as state programs that are not a part of the Medicaid program. Although these programs are critical, they tend to serve a small portion of the long-term-care population. These programs finance about 2 percent of long-term-care expenditures.

Most people receiving long-term care pay for it out of current income and savings. When income plus savings are no longer sufficient, people turn to their state's Medicaid program for financial assistance.[5] As a consequence, Medicaid is the largest single payer of long-term-care services, but direct out-of-pocket expenses are the second most important source of its financing. In 2000 Medicaid accounted for 45 percent of all long-term-care expenditures, 48 percent of nursing-home revenues, and 41 percent of home-care revenues.[6] Families financed 23 percent of long-term care, and payments from families

5. It is believed by some that many middle-income people undertake creative financial planning to appear poorer than they really are in order to gain access to Medicaid sooner. There is little doubt that some of this activity occurs. Certainly, there are legal loopholes that allow such planning, and it is quite likely that state Medicaid programs are somewhat varied in how they administer and enforce their three-year look-back provisions. Studies that have sought to determine the extent of these activities, however, have not yet revealed as much of this type of estate planning as is suggested by the number of attorneys advertising such services (Gruman and Curry 1999; Wiener 1996).

6. National income estimates of private expenditures include home health care only. Because personal care is the bulk of paid long-term care provided in the community, excluding the value of personal or custodial care at home dramatically understates individual out-of-pocket expenditures.

Table 4-1. *Expenditures for Long-Term-Care Services, by Type of Service and Payer*

Billions of 2000 dollars

Payer	Nursing-home care[a]	Home care	Total
Public			
Medicaid[b]	44.4	18.4	62.8
Medicare	9.5	9.2	18.7
Other	2.1	1.7	3.8
Total public	56.0	29.3	85.3
Private			
Insurance	7.4	7.6	15.0
Out of pocket	24.9	6.4	31.3
Other	4.0	1.5	5.5
Total private	36.3	15.5	51.8
Total	92.3	44.8	137.1

Sources: Data from U.S. Department of Health and Human Services (2000); Burwell and Wiken (2001).

a. Nursing-home care includes intermediate care facilities for the mentally retarded. Home care includes home health care, personal care, and home- and community-based waiver services.

b. Medicaid dollars include both federal and state. Home care under Medicaid is primarily provided through home- and community-based waiver programs.

accounted for 14 percent of home-care revenues and 27 percent of nursing-home revenues (table 4-1).[7]

Medicaid

Medicaid expenditures for long-term care have grown substantially in recent years, increasing on average 14.5 percent annually since 1988.[8] However, Medicaid long-term-care expenditures as a proportion of total Medicaid expenditures have declined. In 1988, for example, Medicaid expenditures for long-term care were 44.5 percent of all Medicare expenditures; by 2000, that proportion had fallen to 34.8 percent.[9]

7. Some of this out-of-pocket spending may be attributable to those on Medicaid. Medicaid beneficiaries in nursing facilities are able to retain about $30 a month for their personal needs. The rest of their income, including Social Security and Supplemental Security Income, is turned over to the nursing facility. Some have argued that Social Security and Supplemental Security Income payments to long-term-care providers constitute additional public financing of long-term care. However, in the absence of a nursing-home admission, Social Security or Supplemental Security payments to that individual would be available for personal consumption.

8. Burwell (2000).

9. Burwell and Eiken (2001).

Of the Medicaid expenditures for long-term care, home- and community-based waiver programs have grown the most, increasing nearly 25 percent a year. Expenditures for home health care increased 12.3 percent a year over the decade, and those for personal care increased 9 percent. During this time, nursing-home care expenditures increased, on average, 7.3 percent a year. The pressure to contain the growth of nursing-home expenditures while expanding community-based alternatives has altered the mix only slightly. In 1988, Medicaid nursing-home expenditures were 89.3 percent of all Medicaid long-term-care expenditures. By 2000, Medicaid nursing-home expenditures represented 73.2 percent of Medicaid expenditures for long-term care.[10]

MEDICAID ELIGIBILITY

In general, people who qualify for Medicaid either are recipients of Supplemental Security Income (SSI), defined as "medically needy" under state-specific rules, or have incomes and assets below a state-designated cap. Federal rules entitle elderly and disabled individuals to Medicaid benefits if their incomes and assets are sufficiently low to qualify them for the SSI cash assistance program. In 2000 an individual with a monthly income below $532 and nonhousing assets of less than $2,000 was eligible for SSI.[11] About two-thirds of states permit people to become eligible for Medicaid under "medically needy" programs, which allow them to exclude their medical and long-term-care expenses from their income in determining whether they meet specified income limits.[12]

States also have the option of covering nursing-home care for people whose incomes are below a state-set cap, generally no more than 300 percent of the SSI eligibility level. Individuals who qualify for nursing-home care under Medicaid must contribute all of their income to the cost of their care, with the exception of a small personal-needs allowance of $30 to $90 a month.

MEDICAID "SPENDING DOWN"

People who were not previously covered by Medicaid may become eligible after they have exhausted their resources. Past research on the number of people who obtain Medicaid coverage in this way is generally limited to nursing-home residents, often in one geographical area. One study finds that the community-based spend-down group is larger, younger, and more heavily

10. Burwell and Eiken (2001).
11. Social Security Administration (www.ssa.gov/supplemental-security-income [January 14, 2002]).
12. Schneider, Fennel, and Keenan (1999).

represented by those who are poor or marginally poor than the spend-down population in nursing homes.[13] Spending down among the community-based group appears to have been triggered principally by the cost of acute medical care not covered by Medicare or other third-party payers.

About one-third of discharged nursing-home residents and one-half of current nursing-home residents entered as private-pay residents but spent down to become eligible for Medicaid.[14] Several studies have found that among those who spend down to reach Medicaid eligibility 40 percent do so within a year, and 9 to 16 percent take more than three years.[15] On average, individuals pay $40,000 out-of-pocket for nursing-home care before becoming eligible for Medicaid.[16]

Spend-down rates are closely tied to the length of stay in a nursing home. Among individuals who entered nursing homes as private-pay residents, only 7 percent of those who stayed for less than three months became eligible for Medicaid after exhausting their resources, compared with 55 percent of those who stayed for three to five years. Individuals under the age of 65 are more likely to exhaust their resources than older residents.[17]

Payment patterns for lifetime nursing-home care differ from those for single stays. A study of lifetime patterns of payment among the elderly population finds that 44 percent start and end as private payers, 27 percent start and end as Medicaid beneficiaries, and 14 percent become eligible for Medicaid sometime after their first nursing-home stay. The projected risk of asset spend-down in a nursing home for both elderly users and nonusers is slightly more than 6 percent; and 17 percent of all people who reach the age of 65 are expected to reside in a nursing home and receive Medicaid benefits at some point in the life course.[18]

Spousal Impoverishment

A provision of the Medicare Catastrophic Coverage Act of 1988 protects community spouses of institutionalized individuals from impoverishment. Although the act increased the amount of income and assets that a community spouse is allowed to retain, impoverishment remains a real financial risk. A community spouse is allowed to keep all income received in his or her

13. Temkin-Greener and others (1993).

14. Wiener (1996).

15. Bice and Pattee (1990); Arling and others (1991); Short and others (1992); Temkin-Greener and others (1993).

16. Gruenberg, Alpert, and Burwell (1992).

17. Wiener (1996).

18. Spillman and Kemper (1995, pp. 287–88).

name, but income received jointly must be divided equally between the two spouses. States may set their own income limits but must allow a community spouse to keep at least 150 percent of the federal poverty level for a couple—$1,406 monthly in 2001—but no more than the federal maximum of $2,175. In addition, a community spouse is allowed to keep half of a couple's joint assets but must be allowed to retain at least $17,400 and no more than $87,000.[19]

Although states are required to protect community spouses of Medicaid-eligible nursing-home residents, spousal impoverishment rules are optional for Medicaid waiver programs. Thus community spouses of waiver recipients are often at risk of impoverishment. A substantial number of states (nineteen) do not offer the spouses of waiver recipients the full level of income and asset protection afforded the spouses of nursing-home residents.[20]

MEDICAID BENEFITS

State Medicaid programs must cover nursing-home care and limited home-health-care benefits. States are not required to provide home- and community-based-care services or personal-care services.[21] State Medicaid programs can choose, however, to provide personal care as a statewide benefit or to establish a home- and community-based-care program under a Medicaid waiver.[22] Such waivers allow a state to experiment with specific program designs and target assistance to either a particular category of Medicaid eligibility or a limited area in the state, or both. Like nursing-home residents, waiver recipients must contribute much of their income to the cost of their care. They are allowed to keep substantially more than a nursing-home resident, however. In 1999 the monthly maintenance needs allowance of waiver recipients ranged from $242 to $1,482.[23]

19. Spousal Impoverishment: Section 1924 of the Social Security Act (42 U.S.C. 1396r-5).

20. Kassner and Shirey (2000).

21. Medicaid rules require that nursing-home care and home health care be covered for all eligible program applicants. States also may opt to provide coverage for personal-care services under their Medicaid state plans. In states that choose this option, coverage for services must be available statewide to all eligible applicants. Coverage for services under waiver programs may be limited, however, to specific populations, including those living in specific geographic areas.

22. All states have one or more Medicaid waiver programs, but only thirty states and the District of Columbia have elected to provide statewide personal care to their Medicaid beneficiaries (Doty 2000).

23. Kassner and Shirey (2000).

Medicare

Medicare financed 14 percent of services provided by long-term-care providers in 2000, including 10 percent of nursing-home care and 21 percent of home health care (see table 4-1). Medicare's coverage of long-term care is tied to the need for skilled services.[24] The only nursing-home care covered is that in skilled-nursing facilities (which require a higher ratio of nurses to patients than other facilities) subsequent to a discharge from a hospital. In the case of care at home, where there is often a need for skilled services such as physical therapy, Medicare will cover chronic-care and supportive services incidental to the need for the skilled service. This source of financing is critical to those in need of long-term care; however, the scope of services covered and the duration of services are limited relative to the long-term-care needs of the person.

Private Insurance

Private insurance is similar in this regard to Medicare. Most insurance-financed long-term care is provided in a nursing home or through a home-health-care agency as a part of postacute care or rehabilitation. Financing health care at home or in a nursing home has evolved as a way to reduce hospital costs. Overall, private insurance—including long-term-care insurance—financed about 11 percent of long-term care in 2000 (see table 4-1). A decade earlier, private insurance financed about 2 percent of long-term care.[25] Although some of the increase can be attributed to long-term-care insurance, most of it reflects the intense effort to reduce health-care expenditures generally, and inpatient hospital expenditures in particular, over this time.

Integrating Family and Professionals

Family members and others who are providing care forgo something to provide this care, and therefore there is a cost, certainly to them, their families, and perhaps their employers.[26] In general, families cannot provide all of the

24. There are at least two important exceptions to this. One is hospice care, which may or may not be long-term care, depending on how long the patient lives. The other is the Program of All-Inclusive Care for the Elderly (PACE), which is a joint Medicare and Medicaid program that integrates acute and long-term care for dependent elderly. There are currently twenty-four PACE sites in fourteen states, serving about seven thousand people.

25. U.S. Health Care Financing Administration (1999, table 3).

26. Without knowing the opportunities forgone by each caregiver it is somewhat difficult to estimate the indirect costs of caregiving. Some analysts have used either the

Figure 4-1. *Form of Assistance Received by Community-Resident Adults*
Needing Long-Term Care, 1994

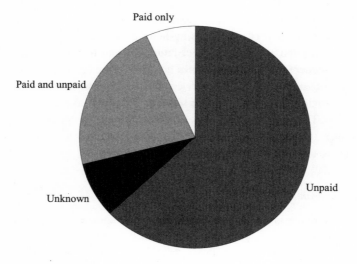

Source: Data from Urban Institute and Congressional Research Service (2000).

care all the time; and even when they do so, they are not necessarily the most appropriate providers.

Families do employ assistance; but relative to the amount of care needed, not much is purchased. Paid direct-care workers working outside of institutions are concentrated in fewer than one-third of all households in need of long-term care. About 7 percent of the adult (aged 18 and older) long-term-care population living in the community relies exclusively on paid assistance, and another 22 percent incorporates paid assistance with unpaid assistance (see figure 4-1).

---

wages of the caregiver or a proxy for such wages; others have used the average wage of direct-care workers to estimate indirect costs. Neither is a satisfactory approach. The latter approach, however, does provide a suggestion of the value of family caregiving. Multiplying the estimated number of hours families provide care by the average wage of direct-care workers, the value of informal caregiving in 1997 was estimated at $196 billion, compared with $83 billion for nursing-home care and $32 billion for home health care (Arno, Levine, and Memmott 1999). However, because families provide care even when paid assistance is provided, this value is surely overstated.

Anticipating the Financial Risk and Consequences of Needing Long-Term Care

Needing long-term care and anticipating that need are two distinctly different states of being. Many of the current problems in organizing long-term care are tied to ways in which long-term care has been financed in the past. A better-funded system with the appropriate mix of services and financial incentives could lead to a vastly better delivery system. The framing of a more rational set of financing arrangements with appropriate incentives for the delivery system goes well beyond the scope of this paper. Instead, the remainder focuses on the financial options currently available to individuals anticipating the need for long-term care. There are not many choices.

There are essentially only three options for anticipating the financial risk of long-term care before the actual need for that care arises. These include moving into an insured continuing-care retirement community, saving for long-term-care services, and purchasing long-term-care insurance. Each approach has its shortcomings, not the least of which is that none of them pools all or even most of the financial risk.

Continuing-Care Retirement Communities

Continuing-care retirement communities are not available everywhere, and perhaps, in terms of culture and life-style, they are not for everyone. There are currently an estimated nineteen hundred continuing-care retirement communities around the country, with about 570,000 housing units.[27] Most of these, however, are not fully insured by the residents of the community. In insured communities, the monthly cost of living in the community to any one resident does not change as they move from independent to dependent living.

Aside from having to move, the biggest obstacle to the continuing-care retirement community is probably the cost. If those in need of such housing could sell their homes and use the proceeds to gain access to a continuing-care facility, then the question would simply be one of location and life-style. The cost of entering such a facility, however, puts it beyond the reach of most people. Continuing-care retirement communities have a nonrefundable entrance fee of about $200,000 (partially refundable entrance fees are three to four times higher) and a monthly cost usually ranging from $2,000 to $2,700. Although in 1998 about 35 percent of all Medicare beneficiaries aged 65 and older had total net wealth in excess of $200,000, only 8 percent had home

27. National Investment Council (2000).

equity of this magnitude.[28] This suggests that for most people the cost of moving into a continuing-care community would substantially exceed their combined home equity and current income.

Saving for Long-Term Care

Saving more is probably always a good idea for most people, unless, of course, they consume less than they need or desire and have no interest in leaving savings to heirs. Assuming one is good at saving for retirement and willing and able to plan also for the contingency of long-term care, how much should one save? Saving for long-term care is not like saving for retirement, for which preretirement income and living expenses can be used to help guide postretirement planning. When it comes to long-term care, one is likely to save either too much or too little, and neither is efficient or satisfactory.

Long-Term-Care Insurance

Purchasing insurance to cover an insurable event seems a more reasonable option than saving for long-term care. Insurance policies essentially prefund the anticipated average expense for a large group of people, in exchange for a fixed monthly payment. However, policyholders' expenses are covered even if their costs exceed the anticipated average: those who require little or no long-term care help finance the cost of care for those who require a lot of care, and so everyone pays the expected average cost. Unfortunately, long-term care insurance does not yet cover the full cost of needed care. Long-term-care insurance is still paying a fixed, predetermined benefit amount. This benefit will certainly help finance the costs of long-term care, and it might fully cover the cost of care, but it is impossible to know, at the time of the purchase, what this cost will be.[29]

There appears to have been a fledgling long-term-care insurance market, in one form or another, since at least the early 1960s.[30] In the mid-1980s, however, several national insurance companies began developing and market-

28. Tabulations of SIPP and AHEAD by the Center on an Aging Society. Estimates of the cost of continuing-care retirement communities were obtained by calling such facilities found through their websites on the Internet.

29. The worst-case situation is that the policy coverage along with other resources is not sufficient to cover needed expenses but is more than enough to disqualify public assistance through Medicaid.

30. Friedland (1990).

ing long-term-care insurance policies nationwide. As states struggled to define and regulate the long-term-care insurance products that were emerging, and with memories of the early years of the development of Medigap policies in the 1960s, the National Association of Insurance Commissioners took a proactive stance and began writing "model legislation" for states to adopt.

According to the Health Insurance Association of America, about 4.1 million persons were insured through long-term-care insurance policies in 1998, compared with 1.7 million in 1992.[31] More than 5.5 million people have purchased a policy at one time or another. This association reports that the average annual premium for long-term-care insurance increased 11 percent between 1995 and 2000, from $1,505 to $1,677, and that the average age of purchasers was 67.[32]

In addition to strengthening consumer protections, federal and state governments have taken a number of actions to promote the purchase of private long-term-care insurance. Very early on, for example, the Internal Revenue Service decided to treat the earnings on premiums collected and held by insurance companies with the same preferential tax treatment that life insurance reserves receive (that is, earnings are not taxed). The Health Insurance Portability and Accountability Act recently extended the tax deductibility of some premiums and tax exemptions for certain benefits to qualified long-term-care insurance policies.[33] Following the enactment of the law, at least nineteen states passed tax credits or deductions for long-term-care insurance policies. As of 1999, some states (for example, Maine, Oregon, and Maryland) also offered tax incentives to employers who contributed to the costs of a group long-term-care insurance plan for their employees.[34]

As of 1998, 29 percent of long-term care insurance policies in force were held through employer-based programs.[35] Employer-sponsored policies offer significant advantages over individual policies, including lower administrative costs, less stringent underwriting, and an efficient mechanism to target younger purchasers. Thus far, relatively few employers have been willing to offer long-term-care insurance to their employees. The Department of Labor estimates that 7 percent of full-time employees in private establishments with one hundred or more employees, and 1 percent of employees in establishments with fewer than one hundred employees, were offered long-term-care plans in

31. Scanlon (2000, p. 10).
32. HIAA (2000, p. 2).
33. Scanlon (2000, p. 12).
34. HIAA (2000, p. 6).
35. Scanlon (2000, p. 11).

1997.[36] In most of these plans, the policyholder pays the entire premium. To date, employee participation rates under these arrangements have been quite low. It is estimated that only 6 to 9 percent of eligible employees take advantage of employer plans when offered.[37]

The first employer to offer long-term-care insurance was the State of Alaska, in 1988.[38] Today, twenty-one states offer private long-term-care insurance to their employees.[39] The largest employer, the federal government, however, is about to offer access to long-term-care insurance to its 2.8 million employees and their parents and to federal retirees. The Office of Personnel Management estimates that as many as 20 million people will be eligible for this insurance.[40] The personnel office anticipates that premiums will be 15 to 20 percent lower than standard premiums because of economies of scale associated with marketing to such a huge group.

Structural Issues Confronting Consumers

That so few people have purchased long-term-care insurance suggests that the products in the market today either do not meet the needs of prospective consumers or are not valued by prospective consumers. There may be a number of reasons: perhaps people do not recognize the risk, or do not value the coverage of that risk at the premium price, or do not see insurance as a preferred option over Medicaid. Of course, consumers may recognize the risk and even want the product but simply be unable to afford it. Either way, it is clear that though versions of private insurance for aspects of long-term care have been around for four or more decades, few people currently have long-term-care insurance.

Long-term-care insurance is now priced like whole-life insurance, charging a level premium based on the age at initial purchase.[41] The younger the age of

36. U.S. Department of Labor (1999).
37. Scanlon (2000, p. 11).
38. Friedland (1990).
39. HIAA (2000, p. 7).
40. Stephan Barr, "Long-Term Care Program Is Unfinished but on Schedule," *Washington Post,* January 16, 2002, Metro section, p. B2.
41. In practice, however, insurance companies have requested and received approval to increase rates on existing policies (Senate Special Committee on Aging 2000). The class action lawsuit *Hanson* v. *Acceleration Life Insurance Company*, which was settled out of court, highlighted this issue: plaintiffs had experienced an approximate 700 percent rate increase in the cost of their "level premium" long-term-care insurance policies between 1989 and 1996. The average age of the plaintiffs was 92.

initial purchase the lower the monthly premiums, because part of the funding of the insurance over time will be derived from the accumulation of the premiums and their tax-free earnings. Benefits are claimed after specific criteria, like the number of limitations and the certified use of specific services, have been met. In this sense, long-term-care insurance resembles disability insurance. As a product, however, it is harder to include in one's financial planning than either life or disability insurance.

Life insurance and, to a limited degree, disability insurance are additive benefits and therefore easier to relate to current and expected earnings. For individuals, these products are primarily intended to cover the financial risks of dying or becoming disabled during one's working years. Knowledge of what Social Security covers and of current and anticipating potential earnings allows prospective policy purchasers to make reasonable guesses as to the amount of life or disability insurance that is needed. Relative differences in risk aversion, discount rates, family formation, and ability to pay are among the reasons people choose different products.

The financial consequences of needing long-term care are not as clear as the potential gap in family income caused by death or disability. The financial risk is more analogous to that of health care: the vast majority of future health-care needs for any one person are not foreseeable. Long-term-care insurance itself, however, is not like health insurance: Health insurance provides asset protection and access to medically necessary care. It is not an indemnity policy providing a fixed level of benefits based on either the severity of the illness or the site of care for that illness.

Prospective purchasers of long-term-care insurance must face a number of decisions: What daily benefit should they select? benefit trigger? waiting period? benefit period? Should the benefit amount increase over time? If so, should that increase be an arbitrary percentage or rather some fraction of the annual change in the consumer price index? All this consumer choice may seem appealing, but how is a potential consumer to know how to evaluate the relation between the choices at hand and what could possibly be needed ten, twenty, thirty, or more years in the future? How does one even compare and contrast alternative versions of policies?

Without question, the risk of needing long-term care increases with age, but individuals' particular long-term-care needs, like health-care needs, will vary at any age. Ironically, though long-term-care insurance is priced like whole-life insurance, the need for long-term-care insurance and the risk of having to use it are the diametrical opposite of those for life insurance. The need for life insurance is probably greatest at the time when the risks are lowest (that is, when the policyholder's children are young).

Undoubtedly as more and more people approach the question of retirement and more and more employers offer and even pay for long-term-care insurance, the number of long-term-care insurance policies sold will grow. As long as long-term care needs can far exceed long-term-care benefits, however, long-term-care insurance will continue to be hard to sell.[42] Based on the growth in this market, it is unlikely that long-term-care insurance will have any appreciable impact on the financing or delivery of care or the long-term-care risks most people face, for at least another generation.

Meeting the Demographic Imperative

The failure to enable people who need long-term care to gain easy access to needed services is, in part, attributable to the failure to pool the financial risks and provide the necessary resources. Unfortunately, long-term-care insurance, as currently structured, has not adequately met the needs of the market. Even if it eventually does so, there is one more critical constraint.

Long-term care is labor intensive. Longer life expectancies and declining fertility rates (since the mid-1950s) will eventually lead to cohorts of older people with relatively fewer adult children upon whom to depend. These same trends in fertility rates have already resulted in a substantial slowing of the rate of growth in the labor force. That a smaller proportion of people, from a shrinking pool of new workers, are choosing employment in nursing, social work, or as direct-care workers has already created a crisis in long-term-care provision.[43] Unless a larger share of people choose to become providers of long-term care, the gap between providers and growing demand will widen. Closing this gap will entail significantly higher costs for long-term care and a reorganization of the way long-term care is delivered.

---

42. Many contend that confusion about Medicare's coverage of long-term care as well as confusion between Medicare and Medicaid has limited the sales of long-term-care insurance. It is true that people are quite confused about Medicare and Medicaid coverage, and it is likely that their confusion has made it harder to sell long-term-care insurance policies. In a recent survey of retirement planning among people in Maryland, however, both purchasers and nonpurchasers of private long-term-care insurance were equally confused about Medicare and Medicaid's role in covering long-term-care needs. Among purchasers and nonpurchasers alike, more than three-quarters (77 percent) were equally misinformed, assuming that Medicare would cover long-term care. On the other hand, purchasers and nonpurchasers were almost equally savvy about the need to expend all of one's resources before becoming eligible for Medicaid. Among purchasers, 49 percent knew Medicaid had an asset test; among nonpurchasers, 47 percent were aware of the asset test (Swamy 2001).

43. Stone and Wiener (2001).

Table 4-2. *Projected Annual Rate of Real Growth in Spending on Long-Term Care from 1998 to 2000*
Percent

Source of financing	Assuming real growth in private insurance coverage	Assuming no growth in private insurance coverage
Medicare	4.0	4.2
Medicaid	2.2	2.9
Long-term-care insurance	9.9	0
Out of pocket	1.4	2.3
Total	3.3	3.0

Source: Author's calculations based on data from CBO (1999) and HCFA (2001).

The gap between supply and demand will not be bridged until the needs of most people using long-term care are met through either long-term-care insurance or the expansion of public programs. The Congressional Budget Office, using the Lewin Long-Term-Care Financing Model, compared simulations of long-term-care financing in 2002 under two alternative conditions of long-term-care insurance coverage: an assumption of substantial growth and an assumption of no growth in private insurance coverage.

Comparing the expenditures by payer, these microsimulations suggest that private long-term-care insurance will lower out-of-pocket expenses for users of long-term-care services but will increase overall long-term-care expenditures. In the absence of any appreciable growth in this insurance coverage, long-term-care expenditures on behalf of the elderly are projected to increase 3.0 percent a year, in real terms, from 1998 and 2020 (see table 4-2). In contrast, if private long-term-care insurance financing increases substantially (almost 10 percent a year), then long-term-care expenditures are projected to increase 3.3 percent annually.

Based on these two competing scenarios, private long-term-care insurance would save Medicare and Medicaid $14.5 billion in expenditures and save users of long-term-care services $9.2 billion. However, the insurance payments for long-term-care services, which would be $36.2 billion, would be greater than the savings to Medicare, Medicaid, and users by more than $12.2 billion. In effect, these simulated scenarios suggest a significant cost shift from Medicaid and Medicare to taxpayers in the form of long-term-care premiums.

Longer life expectancies with a continual decline in fertility rates have already increased the risk and consequences of needing long-term care. Leaders in public policy and private enterprise must first come together to decide what kind of long-term-care system they want for future generations.

References

Alecxih, L. 1997. "What Is It, Who Needs It, and Who Provides It?" In *Long-Term Care: Knowing the Risk, Paying the Price,* edited by Lynn Boyd, 1–17. Washington: Health Insurance Association of America.

Arling, G. W., and others. 1991. "Medicaid Spenddown among Nursing Home Residents in Wisconsin." *Gerontologist* 31 (2): 174–82.

Arno, P., C. Levine, and M. Memmott. 1999. "The Economic Value of Informal Caregiving." *Health Affairs* 18 (2): 182–88.

Bice, T., and C. Pattee. 1990. *Nursing Home Stays and Spend Down in the State of Connecticut: 1978–1983 Admission Cohorts.* Hartford, Conn.: Connecticut Partnership for Long-Term Care.

Burwell, B. 2000. *Medicaid Long-Term Care Expenditures in 1999.* Cambridge, Mass.: Medstat Group.

Burwell, B., and S. Eiken. 2001. *Medicaid and HCBS Waiver Expenditures, FY 1995 through FY 2000.* Resource Network on Home- and Community-Based Services.

Coleman, B. 1996. *New Directions for State Long-Term Care Systems,* vol. 1: *Overview.* Washington: AARP, Public Policy Institute.

Coleman, B., E. Kassner, and J. Pack. 1996. *New Directions for State Long-Term Care Systems,* vol. 2: *Addressing Institutional Bias and Fragmentation.* Washington: AARP, Public Policy Institute.

Congressional Budget Office (CBO). 1999. *Projections of Expenditures for Long-Term Care Services for the Elderly.* Memorandum (March).

Cutler, D. M. 2001. "Declining Disability among the Elderly." *Health Affairs* 20 (6): 11–27.

Doty, P. 2000. *Cost-Effectiveness of Home and Community-Based Long-Term Care Services.* U.S. Department of Health and Human Services.

Friedland, R. B. 1990. *Facing the Costs of Long-Term Care.* Washington: Employee Benefit Research Institute.

Gruenberg, L., H. Alpert, and B. Burwell. 1992. *An Analysis of the Impact of Spenddown on Medicaid Expenditures.* U.S. Department of Health and Human Services.

Gruman, C., and L. Curry. 1999. "Spend-Down Patterns of Individuals Admitted to Nursing Homes in Connecticut." Discussion paper 11-1999. Connecticut Partnership for Long-Term Care.

Health Insurance Association of America (HIAA). 2000. *Who Buys Long-Term Care Insurance in 2000? A Decade of Study of Buyers and Nonbuyers.* Washington (October).

Kane, R. A., R. L. Kane, and R. C. Ladd. 1998. *The Heart of Long-Term Care.* Oxford University Press.

Kassner, E., and L. Shirey. 2000. *Medicaid Financial Eligibility for Older People: State Variations in Access to Home and Community-Based Waiver and Nursing Home Services.* Washington: AARP, Public Policy Institute.

Kaye, H. S., and others. 1996. "Trends in Disability Rates in the United States, 1970–1994." Disabilities Statistics Abstract Number 17. U.S. Department of Education, National Institute on Disability and Rehabilitation Research (November).

Manton, K. G., and X. Gu. 2001. "Changes in the Prevalence of Chronic Disability in the United States Black and Nonblack Population above Age Sixty-Five from 1982 to 1999." *Proceedings of the National Academy of Sciences of the United States of America* 98 (11): 6354–59.

The NewsHour with Jim Lehrer and The Henry J. Kaiser Family Foundation/Harvard School of Public Health. 2001. *National Survey on Nursing Homes.* Health Unit Publication 3171. Menlo Park, Calif. (October).

Scanlon, W. J. 2000. *Long-Term Care Insurance: Better Information Critical to Prospective Purchasers.* GAO/T-HEHS-00-196. U.S. General Accounting Office (September 13).

Schneider, A., K. Fennel, and P. Keenan. 1999. *Medicaid Eligibility for the Elderly.* Washington: Kaiser Commission on Medicaid and the Uninsured.

Short, P., and others. 1992. "Public and Private Responsibility for Financing Nursing-Home Care: The Effects of Medicaid Asset Spenddown." *Milbank Quarterly* 70 (2): 277–98.

Spillman, B., and P. Kemper. 1995. "Lifetime Patterns of Payment for Nursing Home Care." *Medical Care* 33 (3): 280–96.

Stone, R., and J. Wiener. 2001. *Who Will Care for Us? Addressing the Long-Term Care Workforce Crisis.* Washington: Urban Institute and the American Association of Homes and Services for the Aging.

Swamy, N. 2001. "Long-Term Care Insurance: Factors Affecting the Decision to Purchase." Draft, October.

Temkin-Greener, H., and others. 1993. "Spending-Down to Medicaid in the Nursing Home and in the Community: A Longitudinal Study from Monroe County, New York." *Medical Care* 31 (8): 663–79.

Urban Institute and Congressional Research Service. 2000. *Long-Term Care Chartbook.*

U.S. Department of Commerce. Bureau of the Census, Income Surveys Branch. 1993. *Survey of Income and Program Participation.*

U.S. Department of Health and Human Services. 2000. *National Health Expenditures.*

U.S. Department of Labor. 1999. *Employee Benefits in Medium and Large Establishments, 1997.* Bulletin 2517 (September).

U.S. Health Care Financing Administration (HCFA). Office of the Actuary. 1999. *Financing Review* (Winter).

Wiener, J. M. 1996. "Can Medicaid Long-Term Care Expenditures for the Elderly Be Reduced?" *Gerontologist* 36 (6): 800–811.

Commentary on Part One

Comment by Maribeth Bersani

The company I represent, Sunrise Assisted Living, and indeed the entire long-term-care provider industry, has a saying: "Assisted living is changing the way America ages." Actually, America itself has started to age differently, and that is what has brought assisted-living facilities into being. We are all familiar with the changing American demographics: more women are working outside the home; families are smaller; people are living longer; and care for aging or disabled family members increasingly occurs away from home.

As people move into old age, many need assistance with activities of daily living more than they need complex medical treatments. For example, we have seen an increased concern with Alzheimer's disease in our facilities: more people are coming to assisted living looking for outside assistance with the problems created by the disease. This trend toward assistance over treatment has altered long-term-care needs, heightening the demand for assisted-living accommodations.

The consumer preference for residential over institutional care has increased today's options in long-term care. Moreover, consumers themselves are much more demanding and better educated. Better-informed consumers are now demanding a different product when they come looking for long-term care.

The greatest change I see is in the way care is delivered. I first worked in a nursing home in 1972, as an activity assistant. My assignment was to take the residents, most of whom were in wheelchairs, from their rooms and wheel them into the activity room, where some residents played bingo. Few other activities were offered.

Residents are now offered options—not only in recreation but also in everyday activities. They decide when they want to bathe. Locks on residents' doors provide privacy and allow residents to choose when a staff member may enter their rooms. This represents a change in the philosophy of long-term-care provision. We believe in freedom of choice. We believe in letting individuals decide how to spend their time. We recognize the importance of quality of life, not just quality of care.

Progress has also been made in the atmosphere of facilities. In an average assisted-living community today, and even in nursing homes, there is more carpeting than linoleum, fluorescent lights are not used, and corridors are shorter. We in the industry have listened to what consumers want and have responded accordingly, creating more residential and homelike long-term-care environments.

We have come a long way in empowering our elderly population, thanks to the efforts of active ombudsmen. We still have a long way to go, however. As Robyn Stone notes, ageism is still alive and well in the United States. In my professional capacity, I see a form of ageism from regulators and from adult children who think they know more about their parents' needs than the parents themselves. As a result, the elderly are constantly fighting paternalistic attitudes.

We all want our parents to be safe. I worry about my eighty-year-old mother and father. I sometimes wish I could put them in a bubble. I call them when it is snowy and tell them, "Don't go outside, you might slip and fall." I call when it is hot and say, "Don't go outside, you might suffer heat stroke."

But I know that I cannot take control of their lives. I would not want my mother to tell me not to go roller-blading because I might hurt myself. We have to be realistic. We must strive for a balance between safety and choice. We want to provide an environment for our aging population in which they will be safer than at home but one that allows them to live their later years with some degree of autonomy. We cannot tie them up in chairs to keep them safe. Our biggest challenge in this respect is working with regulators and policymakers on this issue. Researchers can help by clarifying the needs and desires of the elderly.

We must guard against the tendency to overreact to reported safety problems in the facilities that care for our elderly, recognizing the importance of the balance between safety and choice. Regulations are important but should not take away resident choice.

Two issues need particular attention. First, I have seen significant improvements in the delivery of long-term care over the past twenty-five years, but innovation has occurred primarily in the private-pay market, and it has not resulted in more affordable options. Second, the quality of care depends in large measure on the quality of the work force. Retention of workers deserves particular attention.

As a number of authors in this volume observe, most people begin to think about long-term care only when a crisis occurs. As providers we need to take responsibility for informing people about their options for long-term care before they are faced with the need for such care. I encourage readers to visit an assisted-living facility and to plan for their later years before such a crisis arises.

Comment by Ingrid McDonald

I represent the Service Employees International Union. The union has 1.5 million members—more than 250,000 of whom are on the front lines in providing long-term care. These include nurse aides in nursing homes, per-sonal-care assistants who visit people in their homes, and a small number of people working in assisted-living facilities. The quality of care provided to the elderly and disabled in long-term care is to a great extent determined by the quality of this work force.

Although recruitment of staff is also a problem, the instability of the work force in long-term care is primarily a problem of retention. Estimates vary widely, but many report staff turnover rates in nursing homes between 80 and 100 percent per year. In a recent survey of 6,991 facilities, the American Health Care Association has found a national turnover average of 76 percent per year.[1] In many states, the majority of certified nurse aides listed in the registries are no longer working in nursing homes. The turnover rate in home health care is probably a little lower than that in nursing homes, but here too we find a transient, unstable work force. If workers could be persuaded to stay, staff problems would be significantly lessened.

The impact of turnover on quality of care is obvious. Some nursing-home residents do not have surviving family, and many never receive a visit from a family member. They create strong bonds with their care providers, and the break in this relationship can be highly stressful, especially for residents with communication impairments. Having to build a rapport with a new provider once, twice, even three times in a year is traumatic for residents and harmful to continuity and quality of care.

What is the cause of this high turnover? I like to call it the WWW problem—wages, workload, and work environment. Long-term care is a low-wage job. The U.S General Accounting Office recently analyzed Current Population

---

1. Health Services Research and Evaluation (2002).

Survey data from 1998 to 2000 and came up with some interesting figures. During that time, this work force was living at or close to the poverty level. One in three aides working in nursing homes earned less than $10,000 a year, and 38 percent reported family incomes below $20,000. Aides working in nursing homes and home health care were twice as likely as other workers to be receiving food stamps and Medicaid, and they were much more likely to lack health insurance: one-third of aides in nursing homes and one-fourth of aides in home health care were uninsured.[2]

Workload is the number-one complaint from nursing-home staff. Workers are sometimes assigned to ten or twelve residents on the day shift and as many as thirty to forty at night. It is simply impossible, physically, mentally, and emotionally, to provide quality care to that many people at one time.

Finally, with respect to work environment, many people talk about the need for a national change in the culture of nursing homes and in all of long-term care. Workers feel that they are not respected and complain that they are excluded from discussions about how care should be provided.

Solutions must be found that address the specific issues of wages, workload, and work environment. Without viable solutions to these root problems, improvement in the quality of long-term care will be difficult to achieve.

Comment by Paul Yakoboski

This discussion focuses on what I label the "reality of paying for long-term care." Roughly 4 percent of long-term-care expenditures are covered by private insurance. Medicare and Medicaid cover about three-fifths, and the rest, one-third or so, is paid for out-of-pocket.

What conclusion regarding private long-term-care insurance should be drawn from this low figure? Christine Bishop notes that insurance does not yet cover much long-term care. The scope and nature of private insurance in the future, she suggests, is unknown. Other commentators would be far less kind, I think, and say, "Well, if we can get only 3.4 million individuals to enroll in private insurance, then this must not be a viable approach to addressing the future long-term-care needs of the baby boomers."

However, I would like to bring a different perspective to this issue and then draw some conclusions from that perspective. First, private long-term-care insurance has been in existence for only about fifteen years. By way of

2. U.S. General Accounting Office (2001).

comparison, 401(k) plans—through which many Americans save for retirement—have been around for more than twenty-five years. Thus long-term-care insurance is a product that can, at best, be described as in its adolescence, and so low current coverage rates should come as no surprise. It is only in the past five years that the market for this product has begun to mature; that is, private long-term-care insurance policies are now offered that have the features, the pricing, and the consumer protections that make them viable, attractive financial products.

Private insurance has great potential to help shoulder more of the load of paying for the long-term-care needs of aging baby boomers. I agree absolutely with Robyn Stone when she says that financing of long-term care will remain a public-private mix. I simply think we need to bring more balance to that mix. Current proportions are greatly out of whack.

I do not view this as an issue of social versus private insurance. Obviously, each has a legitimate role. At the moment, however, social insurance is being asked to carry far too much of the load, and other sources of payment too little. Promoting private insurance will actually strengthen government programs by allowing us to focus scarce public resources where they are truly needed, on those individuals who cannot provide for themselves.

How, then, can private insurance be promoted to help realize its potential? Long-term-care insurance should be positioned as an issue of retirement income security. This is not just catchy marketing by the insurance industry. In 2000, the average yearly cost of staying in a nursing home was $55,000. In a recent survey conducted by the American Council of Life Insurers, 98 percent of survey participants who carry individual policies for long-term care expenses said that is an important part of their retirement planning.

How can this message be delivered to the public? Americans have become fairly well educated about the need to plan and save for retirement. There is no reason that a similar education campaign could not be launched for long-term-care planning, especially if it is packaged as a part of retirement planning.

Who should the messengers be? I think it is the obvious cast of characters that we have relied on in the past: the insurance industry, financial planners, the media, and the government. Substantial resources have already been devoted to planning and saving for retirement income security. It is time to bring long-term-care planning into that picture and make it part of the message, as well.

References

U.S. General Accounting Office. 2001. "Nursing Workforce, Recruitment, and Retention of Nurses and Nurse Aides Is a Grave Concern." Testimony of William Scanlon before the U.S. Senate Committee on Health, Education, Labor, and Pensions (May 17). GAO-01-750T.

U.S. Health Services Research and Evaluation. 2002. "Results of the 2001 AHCA Nursing Position Vacancy and Turnover Survey." American Health Care Association (February 7).

PART TWO

Care for the Elderly and Disabled under the American Social Contract

5

Evolution of the American Social Contract for Care

Theodore R. Marmor

A T THE OPENING of the twenty-first century, Medicare was at the top of the national political agenda but without any clear resolution as to whether it would be changed dramatically, adjusted incrementally, or stalemated politically.[1] The combination of the demands of the presidential race of 2000, the partisan split between the Congress and the Clinton administration, and the ordinary structural constraints of American politics all make the immediate future unclear and longer-term predictions uncertain. What the conflict was about, however, is somewhat clearer. It was a dispute between those who wanted Medicare to remain largely within the confines of the social insurance model of its birth and those who advocated that the program be turned into a voucher scheme. The traditional defenders of Medicare sought to shore up its financial future by committing projected federal surpluses to the program. By contrast, the voucher proponents (using the vocabulary of "premium support") presumed that having Medicare beneficiaries choose among competing health insurance plans was the right course of remedial action.

These were Medicare's reform options before the war in Afghanistan transformed America's political agenda. It is worth emphasizing that competing visions of Medicare's future rest on profoundly different conceptions of the responsibilities and capacities of government in social policy and, in particular, on which social insurance principles ought to apply to the Medicare program. What is equally noteworthy, however, is that long-term care had no obvious place on that agenda—neither during the campaign of 2000 nor in the deliberations of the Breaux-Thomas commission on Medicare's future.

I want here to explore what explains the place—or, more accurately, the absence—of long-term care on the Medicare agenda over the program's

1. Kaiser Family Foundation (1999).

legislative and operational history. That history is crucial for understanding the gap between what Medicare's benefits have been and what policy specialists think they should be. The political history of Medicare (and, in general, its focus on acute care and its avoidance of long-term care and chronic illness) is also important to policy specialists in these areas. Although it focuses on the assumptions that have dominated Medicare's history, this chapter is an indirect but nonetheless important source of lessons for the treatment of long-term-care financing in the United States. The surprises of Medicare's enactment—Part B, on the one side, and a broad Medicaid program, on the other—live with us to this day.

As a first step, I sketch the reform strategy that Medicare represented. From its conceptual origins in the 1950s, Medicare was understood to be a first step toward universal health insurance, and health insurance during that period was overwhelmingly oriented toward financial protection against the costs of acute episodes of illness or injury. So understood, the puzzle is not what conceptions of social insurance prevailed but rather how they bolstered the initial form of Medicare and shaped how it would be expanded. Moreover, Medicare's operational history since 1966 has affected the consideration of long-term care. Since Medicare was implemented in 1966, the aim of universalizing conventional health insurance—and the unexpected role Medicaid came to play in long-term care—effectively foreclosed its expansion into long-term care for most of its history. Finally, the development of procompetitive ideas for public policy during the last half of the 1990s came to play an important role in Medicare debates. As I show in this chapter, that formulation made a bold expansion of Medicare into long-term care even more problematic.

Medicare's Philosophical Roots: Social Insurance and the Presumption of Expansion

The striking fact about the origins of Medicare is not the surprising character of the 1965 program—namely, the unexpected addition of Part B insurance (covering physician care) and the Medicaid program to the hospital insurance proposal requested by the Johnson administration as H.R.1, S.1.[2] Rather, it is the complex evolution of the commitment in the first place to a program for the aged. Hospital insurance for the elderly under Social Security was what reformers thought they could extract from the American politics of the period, not what they ultimately wanted. Medicare proposals thus began with hospital insurance for the elderly, not with the benefits of health insurance it ought to have included (and, in the end, did).

2. This section follows the analysis in Marmor (2000).

The absence of long-term-care coverage in the Medicare legislation of 1965, however, was not a matter of oversight. Long-term care was consciously avoided both in the run-up to 1965 and in legislative deliberations. Instead, Medicare's hospital coverage included a period of posthospital convalescence that was sharply distinguished from the long-term care that the Medicaid program was authorized to finance. Protection from the unbudgetable expenses of acute illness was the announced aim of the Medicare program, but few of its backers imagined that the program features of 1965 constituted reasonable provision of that protection.[3] Rather, in the context of the Great Society's aspirations, the legislation of 1965 was but a first step in a series of pragmatic efforts to make acute medical care universally accessible and its costs more fairly and sensibly distributed across groups, redistributing the financial burdens from the sick to the well and the poorer to wealthier through social insurance taxes. This much is the story I have told in *The Politics of Medicare,* a story that has remained substantially unchallenged since its first telling in 1973.[4]

Appropriate standards of access to services and the distribution of medically related costs are not directly confronted in incremental, pragmatic adjustments to the political possibilities of the moment. The atmosphere surrounding Medicare's enactment was one of great drama and achievement, a big step toward an expanded role of the government in American health insurance. Medicare's philosophical underpinnings—to the extent they were clear in 1965—were largely negative, however, specification of what Medicare was not rather than what its aims and methods fully entailed. So, for instance, Medicare was not to be like the National Health Service of Great Britain, in which medical care is removed from the market and directly provided by public authorities and their contractual agents. That would have been "socialized medicine" for the old, a negative stereotype self-consciously rejected by Medicare's reformers. Nor was Medicare to be "charity" or welfare medicine. Its immediate predecessor—the Kerr-Mills program enacted in 1960—was precisely that and was accordingly judged a great failure. Thus if medical care was to be understood as a merit good and if means-tested programs to ensure its availability were unacceptable, it stood to reason that some other form of government intervention into the medical economy was required. That intervention was health insurance for Social Security beneficiaries on social insurance terms.

With respect to long-term-care coverage, the reasoning was somewhat different. Medicare was conceptualized as governmental provision of conven-

3. Bowler (1987).
4. Marmor (2000).

tional health insurance; socialized health insurance would no doubt have been the most accurate description. The implicit model was the service benefits of Blue Cross, which were primarily aimed at acute medical episodes taking place in hospitals. Long-term care in the 1960s was not part of that conceptual scheme. Indeed, Blue Cross coverage of the period did not include a long stay in a nursing home or extensive home services. Long-term care was conceptualized more as the maintenance of frail persons, with modest or no medical care, the provision of physical security, and what amounted to room and board for those without other options. The fact that Medicaid covered long-term-care benefits—given its means-tested eligibility—was no surprise in the context of American politics of the late 1950s and early 1960s. And that, as we shall see, was fateful for Medicare's development.

The structure of Medicare as enacted—Social Security financing and eligibility for hospital care (Part A), and premiums plus general revenues for physician expenses (Part B)—had a political explanation, not a consistent, clearly understood social insurance rationale. The rhetoric was there, but the public's understanding of the distinctions between social and private health insurance was never deep. The structure of Medicare's benefits themselves, financing acute hospital care and intermittent physician treatment, was not tightly linked to the special circumstances of the elderly as a group. Left out were provisions that addressed the particular problems of the chronically sick (or simply frail) elderly—medical conditions that would not dramatically improve and the need to maintain independent function rather than triumph over discrete illness and injury. Viewed as a first step toward universal health insurance, the Medicare strategy made what seemed like obvious sense. After more than three decades, however, with essentially no serious restructuring of the benefits, Medicare appeared by the mid-1990s philosophically somewhat ungrounded and practically in need of serious adjustment. The program as enacted did not cover the cost of prescription drugs nor extended stays in what we have come to call nursing homes. These omissions—particularly prescription drug coverage—would become major factors in the calls for Medicare reform at the end of the 1990s and remain subordinated on the domestic agenda to the war preoccupations of 2001.

Beyond the continuing mismatch between Medicare's benefits and the health circumstances of many of the elderly, there has always been the unresolved question of what kind of entitlement to medical care Medicare expressed. Medicare's social insurance premises did provide a general basis for a statutory "right" to health insurance coverage. Neither the program's reformers nor subsequent defenders, however, have defined precisely the character of that right or the extent of protection it promised. It is here that the absence of a guiding Medicare philosophy is most apparent. One interpretation of the right to medical care emphasizes, for example, equality of opportunity. For the elderly, circumstances of income, housing, illness, and family all differ, sometimes profoundly. Protection from the expenses of acute medical care, from this point of view, would simply mean that equally ill elderly would receive the same treatment, that their ability to pay for care would be irrelevant to the treatment deemed appropriate. Note that this conception does not require heroic treatment of any particular class of ailments; instead it requires that whatever otherwise appropriate treatment be provided free of the impediments of class, regions, or race. Equal opportunity in this context means equal treatment, not luxurious treatment, heroic treatment, or unlimited treatment. Ascetic equality is no more justifiable than luxurious equality of treatment. Considerations other than equality of opportunity would bear on the extent of treatment equally available.

Medicare's development has not, for example, reflected a clear commitment to this egalitarian conception of the right to medical care. Were it the dominant conception, the United States might well have followed Canada's example and discouraged the independent insuring of medical expenses that Medicare does not bear.[5] Consider, for instance, the way supplementary insurance for the elderly developed. Medicare began with a variety of cost-sharing devices to restrain use, a policy that, in the absence of supplementary insurance, redistributes some of the costs of care to the ill among the elderly. Medicare has a hospital deductible approximating the average cost of one day of American hospital care and a deductible for physician services as well as a coinsurance rate of 20 percent on charges Medicare deems "reasonable." Yet because the incomes of the elderly are unequal, the imposition of equal dollar deductibles or coinsurance inherently places unequal burdens on older Americans of varying incomes.

This situation was further complicated by the 1965 legislative decision to permit supplementary insurance to cover these and other medical expenses. These tax-subsidized insurance policies pay for some of the expenses Medicare does not finance (but typically not long-term care). They regularly finance Medicare's deductibles and coinsurance. More than half of Medicare's beneficiaries had purchased such coverage by the mid-1980s, with the uncovered disproportionately located among lower-income older Americans.[6] As a consequence of this, older Americans face quite different net prices for the care of similar medical conditions. An equal right to health care, properly understood,

5. Evans (1986, pp. 19–24); Marmor and Klein (1986, pp. 25–34).
6. Davis (1985, p. 50).

would proscribe such differences in financing.[7] A policy that expressed such an understanding would either bar the purchase of insurance protection for expenses Medicare does not cover or pay completely for the care deemed medically necessary and fiscally sensible.

The degree to which such reflections have been absent from the deliberations about Medicare helps to explain why, when transformative changes were suggested in the 1990s, the conversations were so confusing and unsettled. For some, breaking up the risk pool of Medicare violated social insurance principles. For others, it is simply a technique for managing public subsidy of health insurance for a particular population.[8]

Another profound question left unresolved in Medicare debates has been whether the program should finance all the medical care passing the test of efficacy or "need," perhaps thereby including long-term care. In the 1980s and 1990s, a number of commentators complained that Medicare's rising outlays unfairly taxed the current working population to produce unwarranted benefits to the contemporary (and often financially comfortable) old. In common language this was the Medicare version of the alleged "generational inequity" of America's social policy toward the elderly. This set of claims raises a number of different issues, only one of which is the topic of reflection here. The most controversial question is whether there are grounds for restricting the care available, even if efficacious and sensible on cost-benefit grounds for the elderly, because of alternative uses of those same funds for other Americans.

This issue highlights claims of generational unfairness that became more prominent as fears about the affordability of an aging population became more widely disseminated in the early 1980s and then again in the late 1990s. Because Medicare and Social Security have always enjoyed broad (if not deeply informed) public approval, many critics have turned to complaints that these popular programs can be neither afforded nor managed. That, in turn, led some thoughtful defenders of Medicare to consider what acceptable constraints on benefits for the elderly might be. Could one, for example, justify the deprivation of effective care for the elderly in a way the elderly themselves might view as just? Note that this sort of discussion effectively precludes discussion of Medicare's expansion—whether for long-term care or prescription drugs. And that is precisely what was the case from 1966 to the late 1990s.

Norman Daniels provided an approach to this question that illuminated the issues at stake in the late 1980s.[9] If one pits the care of an older person against

7. Marmor and Morone (1983).
8. White (1998).
9. Daniels (1988).

that of a younger one, the calculation compares the "utility" of one person to another. This formulation—the interpersonal comparison of utility—is fraught with difficulties no social philosopher has solved. Were the question posed differently, however—comparing benefits over one individual's lifetime—a reasonable case could be made for concentrating more resources earlier rather than later in life. If the right to health care is understood as the right to return to functioning after illness so as to complete one's plan of life, then a more completed life calls for less expenditure—holding illness constant—than a less completed one. The claims of the fifty-year-old, on this account, dominate the claims of the same person at eighty and do so for reasons intelligible to that person. It is as if one were allocating resources over one's lifetime and embodying in that decision a social contract: the older the citizen, the greater the restraint.

This formulation made a genuine contribution to the debate over the allocation of resources for different age groups. It differs from the formulation of generational conflicts in an important respect. The policy of restraint applies not to others but to oneself at a point in the life cycle. The basis is not the gains to us as opposed to the losses of others but the distribution of care to us over time. It is hard to imagine a more important philosophical contribution to debates over Medicare than this distinction between the fair treatment of age and the fair treatment of generations. The treatment of generations takes the accidents of the timing of one's birth to decide who gains and who loses, the very essence of arbitrariness in social policy. The fair treatment of aging—a matter in which all are involved similarly—removes this arbitrariness. Nevertheless, there was a crucial limit on the contribution of such thinking to policy debates over Medicare.

The elaboration about what a just distribution of medical-care resources requires—important as it is for the justification of universal health insurance—can do little to contribute distinctively to a philosophical rationale for Medicare as it stands or how it might be expanded. There was a strategic reason to start government health insurance with aged beneficiaries of Social Security. There was an incremental rationale for extending coverage in the 1970s to those eligible for Social Security's disability program and those suffering from renal failure. That, however, provides neither the grounds for universal coverage nor the special reasons why the elderly should enjoy broader insurance coverage that equally threatened other citizens find impossible to find or afford.

In addition, the special circumstances of Medicare's enactment further undermined the staying power that social insurance principles have displayed, for example, in retirement pensions. From the very beginning, the separate and distinctive financing of Part B benefits—drawn from premiums paid voluntarily (though heavily subsidized) and general revenues—blurred Medicare's link to traditional social insurance sources of revenue. Had Medicare been universalized, the rationalization of its finance would have been more salient. As it happened, the range of financing arrangements gave every theory of public finance a claim on characterizing Medicare. That, in turn, meant there was no single compelling characterization with which to resist alterations or to justify expansion.

There was an organizational counterpart to the waning clarity of Medicare's initial rationale. By that I mean the 1977 shift of Medicare's administration from the Social Security Administration to a newly constituted Health Care Financing Administration. This move seemed to draw Medicare away from its social insurance roots and, at the same time, meant that local offices of the Social Security Administration no longer represented Medicare nor monitored its complexities. In addition, the creation of a comprehensive federal agency reflected the prediction that universal health insurance would happen and that the federal role in medical-care finance should be consolidated. That was, of course, neither the first nor the last time that the conceptions of Medicare adjustments were dominated by ambitious notions of what the larger role of federal health policy would be.

Conceived as a prelude to national health insurance for all, Medicare became one of America's largest social programs, directing enormous medical resources to the elderly and their providers. For a variety of reasons, however, Medicare did not adjust its benefits to the most distinctive medical circumstances of that group: namely, chronic ailments. With all the attention to the future fiscal problems of Medicare in budget debates since the early 1980s, it is particularly noteworthy that there has been relatively little sustained attention to justifying the care the program does and does not finance.

No such discussion took place when the debate over Medicare returned to the center stage of American politics in the period from 1995 to 1999. Instead, what transpired was a fiscal and ideological dialogue that mixed fact with fiction, fear with claimed prudence, and fantasy with sobriety about the future. The result was a debate in 1998 and 1999 that was as detached from the realities of Medicare and the wants of its beneficiaries as had been the debate of 1965 from the understandings of most Americans about what benefits the original legislation covered. In part this gap reflected the absence in America of a guiding philosophy about the proper role of government in medical care, especially an articulation of what health coverage under social insurance required. The lack of clarity became increasingly important as fiscal politics made Medicare's future fearful with forecasts of unaffordability. Viewed this way, understanding Medicare's fundamental presumptions—then and now— is a necessary but not a sufficient prerequisite for anticipating its possible futures. Unless its social insurance roots are reinvigorated, Medicare's programmatic operation will continue to come under pressure to resemble the health insurance practices faced by most citizens. That world is one of competition among managed-care plans whose private regulation of patients and providers had already alienated a majority of Americans by the end of the twentieth century. (Indeed, according to a Harris Poll in 1999, managed care and health insurers were two of the four industries that less than a majority of Americans said they would trust; tobacco and oil were the others.)

Medicare's Constrained Development

Medicare's enactment represented an initial strategic step toward universal health insurance under social insurance premises. The premises, however, were not tightly bound to Medicare's administrative features as they developed, and over time, the philosophical debates over American medicine largely ignored Medicare. As a result, whatever image of Medicare's incremental expansion existed at the outset increasingly lost its force, as the early reformers aged and the understanding of what social insurance required waned. From the stagflation of the 1970s to the economic boom of the 1990s, another set of ideas reshaped the ideological context in which Medicare's political battles were fought. Commonly described as the rise of a procompetitive ethos, this family of notions depended on a set of dichotomies: markets over governments, competition over regulation, individual choice over collective security. These simple formulations, however misleading, became crucial elements of the external environment, setting the terms of the debates over Medicare.

Medicare and the Procompetitive Movement

From our perspective at the start of the twenty-first century, it might seem obvious that the debate over Medicare reform should focus on topics like managed care, competitive health plans, and privatization, to say nothing of prescription drug and long-term-care coverage. Such ideas, however, would have been unthinkable at the time of Medicare's enactment in the mid-1960s. For the quarter century following World War II, American medicine experienced a golden age of medical progress. It was a story of expansion in scientific research, growth of medical institutions, and vigorous efforts to distribute these gains more widely in reforms of the 1960s like Medicare, Medicaid, and the community mental health movement.

In the early 1970s the debates about American medicine shifted in a number of important ways. Claims of crisis became commonplace as stagflation strained American public budgets, the costs of medical care continued to escalate faster than general prices, and the uninsured again received prominent attention. The language of dismay eclipsed the former, celebratory rhetoric. A sense of urgency marked the atmosphere of medical-care debates then, as political élites competed in designing remedies for a medical world that suddenly seemed too costly, too complex, and too callous in an era of rapid inflation and with a growing number of uninsured. At this time it was assumed the necessary tools of reform would be more extensive governmental planning and more vigorous regulation of the costs of care, the quality of clinical practice, and the location and scale of capital investment.

By the end of the 1970s, however, this reformist perspective had been discredited and debunked by many. To promarket critics, the answer to America's medical woes was less regulation, not more, and competitive reforms became a dominant feature of policy debates about American medicine generally.[10] Although Medicare was largely insulated in the 1980s from these newer ideological currents, the genesis of those procompetitive ideas and how they were then applied to American medicine proved crucial to Medicare's fate in the late 1990s and remain important still.

At least three factors made the increased attention to competitive ideas an understandable development in the 1970s. First, traditional concerns about access to medical care and the distribution of its costs began to take a back seat to worries about controlling the costs of care—costs to federal programs, to employers, and so on. Problems of the uninsured and poorly protected could not compete for the public's attention with the genuinely ominous numbers on medical inflation. In 1970, the United States, possessing a strong and growing economy, spent 7.4 percent of its gross national product on health care. In 1980, with a weak economy still reeling from the twin oil shocks of the previous decade, the proportion was 9.1 percent.[11] By 1991 medical care absorbed 11 percent of the gross national product, and by the end of the decade about 14 percent.[12]

A second factor was the general ascendance in academic writing of a particular microeconomic approach to analyzing public policy—or, more accurately, the ascendance of economic analysis that had a deregulatory mission.[13] The antigovernment, free market enthusiasms of economists identi-

10. Marmor (1990).

11. U.S. Bureau of the Census (1990, p. 92).

12. Organization for Economic Cooperation and Development Health Data 2002 (www.oecd.org/EN/links_abstract/0,,EN-links_abstract-684-5-no-no-1125-0,00).

13. It may be hard to rememer, but at one time economics helped to provide justification for government intervention and regulation. The principal motive for increased application for economics to public policy after World War II was the

fied with the University of Chicago conventionally represent this development, but others who would hardly be associated with that movement, like the
Brookings economist Charles Schultze, were also influential.[14] Indeed, it is fair
to say that the neoclassical training of most American economists of this period
made the growth of economic analyses of public policy a factor in this
assumptive shift. All of this provided the intellectual groundwork for making
procompetitive reforms more plausible in medical care.[15]

A third factor bolstering the so-called competitive movement was the
spread of the antigovernment, antiregulatory sentiment to the wider political
arena. Although for many this movement is synonymous with Ronald Reagan's
presidency, it had earlier roots. Richard Nixon's two presidential victories
celebrated the limits of government and the appeal of market competition, even
if his administration's domestic policy actions actually expanded federal social
policy significantly. American commentators often forget the extent to which
Jimmy Carter ran for president on an anti-Washington, antigovernment plat-
form, portraying himself as a down-home farmer who, pitchfork in hand, was
headed to the nation's capital to slay the federal leviathan. The increased
legitimacy of this general political ideology—most obviously consequential in
traditional areas of governmental regulation like trucking, airlines, and finance—made its application to medical care less problematic than would have
been the case at the time of Medicare's birth.

The ideology of competition that arose out of the ashes of the 1970s came
to have considerable political and rhetorical appeal. The simplest version of the
"competitive" answer to social problems was that all public institutions needed
to be restructured to accommodate market incentives. The most zealous
proponents of competition in medical care confidently claimed that a return to
the market would lead to a more sensible control of costs, a more equitable
allocation of scarce medical resources, the creation of a more rational delivery
system, and the delivery of more appropriate (and perhaps better) medical care.
The acceptability of these procompetitive presumptions had become broad
enough by 1980 that the *Report of the President's Commission for a National
Agenda for the Eighties* could unselfconsciously assert that "an expansion of

---

expanding of government as a purveyor of large public programs entailing major
expenditures (Melhado 1988, p. 35).

14. Melhado (1988, p. 145).

15. Indeed, Evan Melhado cites a personal telephone conversation in which the
Stanford economist Alain Enthoven reports that he had read Schultze's book, *The Public
Use of Private Interest*, shortly before devising his Consumer Choice Health Plan and
that he regarded his own book as the "working out" in the health care economy of an
example of Schultze's general propositions (Melhado 1988, p. 37).

the role of competition, consumer choice, and market incentives rather than government control is more likely to create the much needed stimulus toward greater efficiency, cost consciousness, and responsiveness to consumer preferences so visibly lacking in our present arrangements for providing medical care."[16] Similar claims received widespread coverage in trade journals, in the popular press, and on Capitol Hill.[17]

The legacy of the debate over medical-care reform since the 1970s, from the standpoint of this discussion, is threefold. On the one hand, the case for an American version of national health insurance—a Medicare program for all, for example—was weakened. In fact, critics used the problems of American medicine to condemn governmental incapacity. On the other hand, promoters of competition in medicine compared idealized dream worlds with real systems (and, unsurprisingly, ideal systems seemed preferable on paper). To persuade the public of the creditability of the imagined market world, the language of health debates was shrewdly altered. The vocabulary and terminology of economists became the vernacular, and the unquestioning use of this jargon became much more pervasive in debates.[18]

In place of national health insurance, the Clinton reform effort left a stalemated political outcome—symbolized by the literal disappearance of the Clinton plan in September 1994—followed by an unprecedented pace of change in American medical-care arrangements ever since. Although this is not the place for any extended discussion, it is important for this assessment of the role of competition to note whatever connections there were between the long buildup of competitive ideas and the Clinton debacle.

The resulting story was one of great hopes, great changes, and great disappointment. The hopes of some of the procompetitive advocates—of either consumer sovereignty or organizational reform—were a combination of universal coverage and competitive conditions in the pricing and delivery of medical care. The Clinton reformers also hoped to combine competition in the delivery of care with egalitarian financing of the basic insurance. Their hopes, as we know, were dashed completely. Yet the story was more significant than that. By capturing the interests and energies of so many reform actors, the procompetitive movement siphoned energy away from other strategies of reform in American public life.

The legacy of this rise and transformation of competitive ideas in medical care will be with America for decades to come in the twenty-first century.

16. President's Commission for a National Agenda for the Eighties (1990, pp. 78–79).

17. See, for example, Christianson and McClure (1979) for trade journals and Demkovich (1980) for coverage in the popular press and on Capitol Hill.

18. Marmor (1998).

Without the regulation proposed by the Clinton plan, the advocates of so-called managed competition were set loose. By 1996, 70 percent of Americans were in insurance plans that are characterized as "managed care." Most of those plans manage little else but costs, and in doing so, they restrict the choices of both medical professionals and their patients. In the name of expanding choice, American medicine went through a period of extraordinary reduction of choice. Aggregate health costs rose at lower rates in the mid-1990s, but that fact can be misleading. The ratio of medical-care inflation to general inflation, for example, was not markedly reduced. The rise in costs to American firms did slow for a time, however, with the externalizing of more costs—both fiscal and psychic—to patients and providers.

Finally, there has been enormous change in the ownership and behavior of insurers, hospitals, medical plans, and drug firms. Organizational consolidation describes much of what has transpired: the growth of multihospital chains like Columbia HCA and the spread to nationwide activities of prepaid group-practice organizations like Kaiser Permanente. In addition, there has been a shifting of financial risk—as with carving up capitation payments—and the creation of new firms less to manage medical services than to constrain what care can be given and to reduce or slow the rate of growth in the prices paid.

All of this constitutes an extraordinary set of ironies. In the name of competition, choice narrowed. In the name of consumer responsiveness, consumer complaints shifted in character and increased in anger. In the name of American entrepreneurialism, American physicians turned into employees of firms owned by others. Choice without change, change without choice—this captures the ironies. The politics of medicine, as a result, will be increasingly fought out in state legislatures.[19] There the disputes are over how much public regulation there should be over the enormous amount of private regulation that has already transpired. Few observers would have predicted the subject of controversy in the state legislatures of the mid-1990s: issues like drive-by mastectomies, limits of one day's hospitalization for the delivery of a child, or gag rules on what doctors could tell their patients about the limits of their managed-care plans. Procompetitive enthusiasts did not predict such disputes either, but in part they arose because of the role such ideas play in the complicated politics of American medicine.

Since the 1970s there has been a constant and broad dispute over the proper role of government in capitalist democracies. The arguments in favor of increased competition—in medical care generally and particularly within health insurance—received far more favorable responses than at any other time

19. See Rich and White (1996).

since World War II. The United States responded to this differently from other industrial democracies. In Europe the argument for increased competition overwhelmingly took for granted that universal entitlement to health insurance was a given. American arguments over the role of competition were part of the broader disputes over whether universal health insurance coverage was desirable and could be implemented. As a result, the story is the rise of procompetitive ideas without the counterpart of guaranteed insurance coverage.

The third legacy of the politics of Medicare (and major medical reform) is that expansion of the program into long-term care has never really gotten serious attention. The development of Medicaid presented a means-tested option for those whose long-term-care expenses caused poverty.[20] The crucial point is that the availability of Medicaid reduced the demand that Medicare attend to the problem of frailty in the absence of acute illness. Moreover, the realities of how Medicaid is administered means that in many states it has been a program of long-term care, supplementing Medicare for families for which spending down produces financial eligibility. The combination of antigovernment sentiments and skepticism about the health insurance coverage of the elderly under contemporary Medicare weakened the appeal of reformers seeking to improve Medicare. Even in the context of expansionary talk about Medicare, the object has been prescription drugs, not long-term care, in most instances. For all of these reasons, an expansion of Medicare into long-term care—along the lines, for example, Bob Ball suggested in his book some ten years ago—will require a major shift in the political landscape.[21]

20. The story of Medicaid's expansion of long-term care financing from its legislative birth in 1965 has been told many times. What is less well known is when and how Medicare flirted with financing long-term care over time. At the outset of the program in 1966, the only concession Medicare made to long-term care services—whether nursing home care or home- and community-based services—was posthospital convalescence and home health visits devoted to rehabilitation. This, of course, simply illustrates the acute care focus of the original Medicare program. That changed for a time in the late 1980s and early 1990s, as one of the long-term care experts, Joshua Wiener, has clearly argued. "Court decisions," he noted in 2001, changed this firm avoidance of chronic care, and "Medicare's home health benefits became much more oriented . . . to long-term care during the 1990s . . . , with expenditures increasing eight-fold between 1988 and 1997." At the same time, Medicare's nursing home benefits increased dramatically during this period, prompting substantial policy concern and reimbursement changes. As Wiener rightly notes, "Medicare benefits are now [2002] less long-term care oriented than they were just a few years ago" (Wiener 2001, pp. 88–89). This sketch is an exception to the general Medicare portrait of this chapter; it is not news to the long-term care specialists but may be to the wider Medicare community.

21. Ball (1989).

References

Ball, Robert M. 1989. *Because We're All in This Together: The Case for a National Long-Term Care Insurance Policy*. Washington: Families USA Foundation.

Bowler, M. K. 1987. "Changing Politics of Federal Health Insurance Programs." *Political Science* 20 (2): 202–11.

Christianson, J. B., and Walter McClure. 1979. "Competition in the Delivery of Medical Care." *New England Journal of Medicine* 301 (15): 812–18.

Daniels, Norman. 1988. *Am I My Parents' Keeper: An Essay on Justice between the Young and the Old*. Oxford University Press.

Davis, Karin. 1985. "Access to Health Care: A Matter of Fairness." In *Health Care: How to Improve It and Pay for It*. Washington: Center for National Policy.

Demkovich, L. E. 1980. "Competition Coming On." *National Journal* 12 (28): 1152.

Evans, R. G. 1986. "Finding the Levers, Finding the Courage: Lessons from Cost Containment in North America." *Journal of Health Politics and Law* 11 (4): 585–615.

Kaiser Family Foundation. 1999. "Voters Say Medicare Top Health Issue for New Congress." In *Post-Election Survey: Priorities for the 106th Congress* (January 14).

Marmor, T. R. 1990. "American Health Politics, 1970 to the Present: Some Comments." *Quarterly Review of Economics and Business* 30 (4): 32–42.

———. 1998. "Hope and Hyperbole: The Rhetoric and Reality of Managerial Reform in Health Care." *Journal of Health Services Research and Policy* 3(1): 62.

———. 2000. *The Politics of Medicare*. 2d ed. Aldine de Gruyter.

———. 2001. "How Not to Think about Medicare Reform." *Journal of Health Politics, Policy, and Law* 26 (1): 107–17.

Marmor, T. R., and Rudolf Klein. 1986. "Cost versus Care: America's Health Care Dilemma Wrongly Considered." *Health Matrix* 4(1): 19–24.

Marmor, T. R., and J. A. Morone. 1983. "The Health Programs of the Kennedy-Johnson Years: An Overview." In *Political Analysis and Medical Care: Essays,* edited by T. R. Marmor. Cambridge University Press.

Melhado, E. M. 1988. "Competition versus Regulation in American Health Policy." In *Money, Power, and Health Care*, edited by E. M. Melhado, Walter Feinberg, and H. M. Swartz. Ann Arbor, Mich.: Health Administration Press.

President's Commission for a National Agenda for the Eighties. 1990. *Report of the President's Commission for a National Agenda for the Eighties*. U.S. Government Printing Office.

Rich, R. F., and W. D. White. 1996. "National Health Reform: Where Do We Go from Here?" In *Health Policy, Federalism, and the American States,* edited by R. F. Rich and W. D. White. Washington: Urban Institute Press.

U.S. Bureau of the Census. 1990. *Statistical Abstract of the United States, 1990*. U.S. Government Printing Office.

Wiener, Joshua M. 2001. "Country Portrait: USA." Paper prepared for Four Country Conference on Aging and Health Policy, Ottawa, Canada, July 12–14.

White, Joseph. 1998. "'Saving' Medicare: From What?" Paper prepared for the Annual Meeting of the American Political Science Association, Boston, September 3–6.

6

Medicare Coverage for Chronic Conditions: The HIV-AIDS Example

Chris Collins and June Eichner

MEDICARE PRESENTLY SERVES 34.4 million elderly and 5.5 million disabled persons under the age of 65. Nearly all of the disabled beneficiaries and 82 percent of the elderly beneficiaries have at least one chronic condition. Although Medicare has never fully covered the range of services needed by those with acute-care needs, its gaps are even more apparent to those with serious chronic conditions.

In 2000 the National Academy of Social Insurance, together with the National Association of People with AIDS, examined the role of Medicare in its provision of care for persons with chronic conditions, using HIV-AIDS (human immunodeficiency virus–acquired immunodeficiency syndrome) as an example of a chronic condition. This research study assessed the experience of Medicare beneficiaries with HIV-AIDS, including Medicare's gaps in coverage, their need for supplemental insurance, and the coordination and information issues they face. It also examined the benefits-counseling programs that some HIV-AIDS organizations have developed to help their clients piece together a synthetic health coverage "system." The experience of the HIV-AIDS population provides lessons for other chronic-condition populations and should increase the understanding of policymakers grappling with the design of Medicare benefits and coverage, as well as the coordination of services across various public and private payers.

The study was conducted in California, a state with a high prevalence of HIV infection, a diverse patient population, and a variety of community-based models and resources available to people with HIV-AIDS. Study components included a series of structured interviews and a review of federal, state, and local program regulations. Respondents to the interviews included regional staff of the Health Care Financing Administration (now known as the Centers for Medicare and Medicaid Services) and the Health Resources and Services Administration, state officials, field staff of the Social Security Administration, local welfare agencies, AIDS and aging organizations, and physicians and other service providers.

Although the experiences of people with HIV-AIDS are in some ways unique, they provide a window into the future of the Medicare population. Like many elderly beneficiaries with long-term chronic illnesses, HIV patients receive much of their health care outside of the hospital and are heavily dependent on expensive prescription drugs that are not covered by Medicare. The experiences of people with HIV-AIDS illustrate the complex care-management needs that are also becoming increasingly common among older Medicare beneficiaries. As with other disabled Medicare beneficiaries under the age of 65, the number of beneficiaries living with HIV-AIDS is expected to increase significantly as drug therapy transforms the disease into a long-term chronic condition. Such beneficiaries will most likely live with the disease for many years but will also have significant chronic-care needs.

The Role of Medicare in HIV-AIDS Care

Medicare is a major payer for HIV-AIDS services. Approximately one in five adults who are receiving regular care for HIV are enrolled in Medicare. In fiscal year 2000, Medicare spent approximately $1.7 billion to care for people with HIV-AIDS. From 1995 to 2000, Medicare expenditures for people with HIV-AIDS grew by 70 percent. More than one-fourth of federal spending on HIV-AIDS care is from Medicare.

Despite Medicare's large role in payment for HIV-AIDS services, there is little awareness of the role that Medicare plays in providing services to people with HIV-AIDS. Medicare is largely viewed as a program for the elderly (who constitute 87 percent of the Medicare population). Respondents to the interviews conducted in connection with this study felt that disabled beneficiaries under the age of 65 do not receive the same attention as aged Medicare beneficiaries and that disabled beneficiaries with chronic conditions (such as HIV-AIDS) receive even less attention than beneficiaries with "classic" disabilities (for example, mobility problems).

Respondents who knew of the Medicare program and the range of services it pays for appreciated the role it played in their clients' lives. Many said that Medicare coverage fills a large share of the insurance gaps for those who have lost their individual or employer-sponsored insurance after they were no longer able to work. For those who depended on Medicaid before becoming eligible for Medicare, Medicare allows them to receive care from physicians in private practice, as few private practice physicians are willing to provide care to beneficiaries with only Medicaid coverage.

Gaps in Medicare Coverage

Social Security and Medicare eligibility guidelines do not provide benefits to many persons with HIV. Clinical guidelines call for regular care from a physician early in the course of HIV infection. However, to qualify for Medicare, a person must be deemed by the Social Security Administration to be permanently disabled (defined as unable to work). Once disability has been determined, Medicare coverage does not begin for another twenty-eight months. Respondents said that it is illogical to withhold coverage until a person is severely disabled, that it makes much more sense to provide coverage to delay the progression of the disease.

People with HIV-AIDS who become eligible for Medicare find that it does not pay for a significant share of their health-care needs. Medicare's gaps include its infamous lack of prescription drug coverage—crucial therapy for people with HIV-AIDS. Medicare also has inadequate coverage or lack of coverage for services vital to the care of HIV-AIDS beneficiaries, including mental health services, case management, community-based care, and a variety of other support services.

Because of the gaps in Medicare, beneficiaries must find other programs to help pay for their health-care services. As beneficiaries seek supplemental health coverage, they find that though there are numerous potential benefit and insurance options, the rules are complex and often conflicting. The virtual alphabet soup of programs available makes for a fragmented and complex payment and care system.

The major programs and insurance used by beneficiaries include California's Medicaid program (Medi-Cal), AIDS Drug Assistance Program, private insurance, Medi-Cal HIPP (Health Insurance Premium Payment), and CARE-HIPP (supported by the Ryan White CARE Act). Some are available to enrollees without regard to health status (for example, employer-sponsored insurance); others are designed specifically for those with a high-cost disease (for example, Medi-Cal HIPP); several are available only to people with HIV-AIDS (for example, CARE-HIPP and AIDS Drug Assistance Program). According to benefits counselors, most of the Medicare enrollees they advise are successful at finding supplemental insurance that meets a large share of their health-care needs.

Coordination and Information Issues

The complexity of Medicare's interaction with other health coverage programs accentuates the need for coordination among agencies and increases the

demand for information. The lack of coordination among payers and programs, however, makes it less likely that information is shared across agencies
and staff.

The search for comprehensive health coverage is further complicated by the
fact that each program is separately administered, with different eligibility
requirements and application processes. Staff members of each program and
agency know little about other programs, and so they are often unable to help
coordinate coverage. Because disabled persons gain access to Medicare by
applying for disability insurance at their local Social Security Administration
offices, and because the agency is in charge of Medicare eligibility, many return
to the Social Security office with their Medicare questions. Social Security staff,
however, lack information about how Medicare works and where beneficiaries
can get information about it. They claim that the Centers for Medicaid and
Medicare Services (CMS) have not been interested in training them. In fact, one
CMS regional staff told us that the staff at the Social Security Administration
does not need to know about Medicare because "Medicare is CMS's job."

Interagency coordination is limited and is a problem when beneficiaries
receive coverage through many different agencies and programs. The multiple
programs are administered by different agencies. For example, Medicare is
administered by the CMS, whereas the AIDS Drug Assistance Program is
administered by the Health Resources and Services Administration and the
State of California. In addition, some programs are managed by separate
divisions within an agency. For example, Medicare and Medicaid are run by
different divisions of the CMS's central and regional offices. (Medicaid is also
administered by the state and counties.) We heard that staff at the numerous
agencies do not talk with one another and do not have systems in place to
facilitate communication of changes in program eligibility and benefits. We
were told that agency staff and the community-based organization staff need to
be cross-trained in each other's programs. As one benefits counselor said, "It
is not enough to know a single program; staff must understand the big picture
to help clients piece together comprehensive coverage."

All of our respondents said that they and their clients find Medicare to be
confusing and complex. There is confusion about the difference between Parts
A and B. Moreover, before applicants become eligible for Medicare, they
receive cards in the mail with instructions to send the card back if they do not
want Part B. A number of respondents told us that their clients misunderstand
the instructions, return the card, and as a result, inadvertently decline Part B
coverage. Beneficiaries also are confused about how much of their bills are
covered by Medicare, what benefits are covered, how Medicare coordinates
payment with other coverage, and which providers are available to them.

Despite the need, Medicare information is difficult to access. Medicare information from the CMS is provided through its booklet for beneficiaries, "Medicare and You." According to respondents, the booklet is helpful to better-educated clients, though it is mailed out once a year to all beneficiaries. Because the mailing is not timed to coincide with enrollment, a new beneficiary could wait nearly a year to receive the information. The CMS also supports a Medicare toll-free hotline and the State Health Insurance Assistance Program, but few of our respondents were aware of these resources. According to respondents, these resources are targeted to elderly beneficiaries and not to disabled beneficiaries under the age of 65.

To address these issues, a number of AIDS organizations have created staff positions devoted specifically to benefits counseling. Benefits counselors are instrumental in providing information and advice on Medicare, Social Security, and other health and income programs; assistance in filling out eligibility forms; advocacy and appeals; coordination of benefits; and building relationships with local Social Security Administration, welfare, state, and other office staff. According to respondents, the role of benefits counselors is crucial. In addition to assisting their own clients, they provide education, training, and assistance to staff at other community organizations.

Conclusion

Policymakers and staff at the Centers for Medicare and Medicaid Services, other federal and state agencies, and chronic-disease and aging associations will need to work together to address the following Medicare issues: an incomplete benefits package; complicated rules and regulations; insufficient information about Medicare and its coordination with other payers; lack of coordination of eligibility requirements and benefits; lack of coordination among agencies and staff; insufficient attention to the disabled population under the age of 65; and insufficient support and funding for benefits counselors. A number of respondents also expressed the view that the solution to the problem of coordination of coverage would be a national health program.

There are important lessons about the provision of long-term care to be learned from the experience of California's HIV-AIDS community, although policymakers should be aware that the great majority of Medicare beneficiaries with chronic diseases have even less access to supplement program and counseling supports than do people with HIV-AIDS. People living with HIV are a relatively young and well-organized chronic-disease population that has successfully lobbied for additional programs and regulations to support their health coverage. In addition, communities such as San Francisco and Los

Angeles have long-established HIV-AIDS community-based providers and organizations, and their medical and social support systems are considered among the most advanced in the United States. Thus the experiences of California beneficiaries with HIV-AIDS described here are a best-case scenario; in much of the nation and for those with other chronic conditions, the situation can be even more difficult. Nonetheless, the lessons learned from this population should well serve Medicare beneficiaries with other chronic conditions.

Commentary on Part Two

Comment by Michael Hash

The presenters in this section have made a compelling case that Medicare's design and most of its policies do not match the needs of today's seniors and people with disabilities. Of course, as Ted Marmor's paper makes clear, Medicare was not really designed initially to meet the long-term-care needs of its beneficiaries. In fact, Marmor makes an important point in terms of the historical roots of Medicare by saying that long-term care was viewed then, and to some degree is viewed now, as a benefit that should be means-tested as opposed to being a part of a social insurance program to which all have access.

The original concept of Medicare was based on the current model for employment-based health insurance, which has been in place since the mid-1960s—most particularly, the insurance that federal employees had at that time. Medicaid, something of an afterthought in 1965, has taken on the burden of providing most nursing-home care to those who are impoverished, and, of course, that coverage has led to a strong institutional bias for care of the frail elderly and those with disabilities.

Now, of course, we inhabit a very different world, with longer life spans, longer periods of coping with the consequences of often multiple chronic diseases, and the lack of coverage, both private and public, for the kind of functional assistance that is a prerequisite for maintaining independence and maximizing the quality of life. Current policies, particularly across Medicare and Medicaid and private insurance, are fragmented, and those with chronic conditions often find it difficult to navigate the world of long-term-care services.

Chris Collins and June Eichner's case study makes a compelling point about the failure of Medicare to serve the vast array of needs of individuals who are faced with chronic diseases, particularly a disease like HIV-AIDS. Although most people think that Medicare's failure to cover prescription drugs is the major issue, that Medicare does not provide support for care coordination, care planning, care assessment, and care integration is, to my mind, equally problematic, especially for people who have one or more chronic diseases.

During my time with the Health Care Financing Administration (HCFA), now the Centers for Medicare and Medicaid Services (CMS), we struggled with how to reshape the existing public programs to better meet the needs of beneficiaries with long-term-care needs. We made fairly limited and marginal progress. Without a substantial redesign of these programs, I do not think much further progress can be made. State Medicaid waivers have become essential tools in expanding home- and community-based services to help extend independence and to give people choices in how they receive their support for long-term care—either in an institutional setting or in a home- and community-based environment.

Our work was reinforced by the Supreme Court's *Olmstead* decision, which requires that people with disabilities be offered opportunities to be treated in the least restrictive settings. This decision has propelled the states' movement into more home- and community-based service options for people with disabilities.

Unfortunately in today's fiscal environment, having moved from surpluses as far as the eye can see to deficits almost as extensive, it is going to be much more difficult to make the kind of progress in long-term-care support that is needed. Clearly, the CMS's effort to work on demonstration projects involving those with dual eligibility has not gone as far as it should. It foundered on the shoals of two problems: how much of the long-term-care payment for dual eligibles should Medicare take on, and who should control those streams of funding for long-term care.

Several promising ideas and opportunities can help create a more coherent course for long-term-care support. First and foremost, we need to stop focusing exclusively on payment systems and think about designing a delivery system that works best for the beneficiaries who need the support. Only when that is in place should we be addressing payment design. Otherwise we are putting the cart before the horse.

We should begin to think about how to get more information to consumers about provider performance. As Tom Scully notes in the epilogue to this volume, performance indicators and the dissemination of them will help to inform the public and give people the tools to make more informed judgments about the quality of care they might receive for various long-term-care services. Moreover, it is time to begin a more comprehensive review of the private insurance market for long-term-care insurance. We need to know how the tax provisions extending favorable tax treatment to private long-term-care policies under certain conditions have changed the market.

I suggest further promotion of dual-eligibility demonstration programs and waivers to see whether there is an opportunity to serve this population more effectively. Finally, a host of Medicare modernization proposals would permit Medicare to support care assessment, care planning, and care coordination, including support for disease management. In adopting these policies for Medicare it is particularly important to take account of the needs of individuals with multiple chronic conditions, which is more typical than isolated single chronic conditions in the Medicare population today.

These reforms could help us move the coordination of long-term-care services forward and better meet consumers' needs. Their implementation, however, will be challenged by our currently constrained budget resources.

Comment by Shelley I. White-Means

As was frequently noted during the conference on which this volume is based, the long-term-care system has no coordination through provider markets. Older persons are not aware of the diversity of services that are available, how to obtain those services, how much services cost, whether subsidies are available for those services, and which service is better than another. Thus the task for their families is to piece together the various services to develop something that resembles a complete care plan. This is a serious problem in our long-term-care system, and it requires an immediate solution—possibly even, as Ted Marmor suggests, a change in the political climate.

Other misalignments occur because of three factors. First, there are racial disparities in older persons' use of acute-health-care services.[1] Thus Medicare does not ensure equality of opportunity in health-care utilization. Second, poverty restricts the access of many older persons to the services they need. Third, the multifaceted role of caregivers receives far less attention, and support, than its importance to long-term care warrants.

Older African Americans who live in the community are more likely to report incidents of medical conditions and disabilities than whites. Thus we find more reports of joint conditions, glaucoma, diabetes, high blood pressure, and cognitive disorders. Yet blacks are less likely than whites with similar medical conditions to use acute-care services, particularly prescription drugs and physician services.[2] Even research that controls for differences in income, insurance coverage, and education cannot fully explain why black older persons underutilize acute-care services.

1. Mayberry, Mili, and Ofili (2000); Waidman and Rajan (2000); Weinick, Zuvekas, and Cohen (2000).
2. White-Means (2000).

Why do I emphasize acute care, when the primary focus of this conference is on long-term care? When there are problems in access to acute care, there will also be problems in access to long-term care. Researchers point to three characteristics that limit access to acute-care services: availability, accessibility, and acceptability.[3] Residential segregation and geographic distribution of facilities create structural barriers to access. Access problems also arise when patients lack the knowledge and networks for obtaining information. In addition, patient perceptions of unfavorable and possibly culturally insensitive doctor-patient interactions can discourage them from seeking the services they need.

The gap in the provision of acute-care services, especially in the use of physician services, has important implications for the care of African American and Hispanic older persons. If health-care systems lack incentives to deliver a coordinated mix of services to older persons, then physicians serve a central role as gatekeepers who identify and certify eligibility for community services.[4] Because blacks and Hispanics underutilize physician services, they lack access to those gatekeepers who could assist them in developing the mix of community services.

Continuing-care retirement communities, long-term-care insurance, and saving are some of the options available for long-term care. Low income, however, is a significant barrier to these three avenues as feasible options for many older persons. African American and Hispanic older persons stand in unique positions of deprivation. According to the National Center for Health Statistics, black and Hispanic older women are two and a half times more likely, and black and Hispanic older men four times more likely, than their white counterparts to be impoverished:[5]

Race	Women	Men
White	11.5	5.6
African American	28.8	21.8
Hispanic	26.3	20.3

This suggests that among older blacks and Hispanics, there is a significant dependency on Medicare and Medicaid and also limited private sources of funding for long-term care.

---

3. Wallace (1990).
4. Cohen and others (1997).
5. Kamarow and others (1999).

A final critical part of the misalignment relates to the caregivers. Caregivers are an important part of the financing of long-term care. The long-term-care system functions because its unpaid informal caregivers (family and friends) are there. The uncompensated cost of caregiving hours in dollar terms is about $196 billion, exceeding total expenditures for nursing homes and home-health-care agencies.[6] Yet reported costs of caregiving are underestimates because they exclude some costs that are difficult to measure.

A recent MetLife study notes, for example, that employer-related annual productivity losses owing to caregiving were $11.4 billion to $29 billion in 1997.[7] Another MetLife study estimates that caregivers are forfeiting about $659,000.00 a person, on average, in lost wages, Social Security benefits, and pension contributions because they are decreasing their work hours, taking less demanding jobs, and retiring early.[8] In addition, I suspect that long-term care is being financed through the declining health, both physical and mental, of caregivers. Good measures of the health costs of caregiving are lacking, however; conclusions await the results of current research efforts.

Thus an accounting of the costs of long-term care should also include lower work-force productivity, the depletion of the current and future financial resources of caregivers, and exhaustion of current health and mental well-being of caregivers. Moreover, the financing of long-term care through caregivers varies by race and ethnicity. Ethnic-minority older persons rely more heavily on informal caregivers (that is, they receive more hours of caregiver support); their caregivers are more likely to be in the sandwich generation and less likely to leave the labor market because of these responsibilities.[9] Are we depleting vital future resources by financing the care of older persons with caregiver services?

References

Arno, Peter, Carol Levine, and Margaret Memmott. 1999. "The Economic Value of Informal Caregiving." *Health Affairs* 18 (2): 182–88.

Cohen, Robin, and others. 1997. "Access to Health Care, Part 3: Older Adults." In *Vital and Health Statistics: Data from the National Health Survey,* ser. 10, no. 198. Hyattsville, Md.: U.S. Department of Health and Human Services, Centers for Disease Control and Prevention, National Center for Health Statistics.

Dessoff, Alan. 2001. "Caregiving Burdens Hit Low-Income and Minority Boomers the Hardest." *AARP Bulletin* 42 (8): 6.

6. Arno, Levine, and Memmott (1999).
7. Metropolitan Life Insurance Company (1997b).
8. Metropolitan Life Insurance Company (1997a).
9. Dessoff (2001); White-Means and Thornton (1990a and 1990b).

Kramarow, Ellen, and others. 1999. *Health and Aging Chartbook: Health, United States.* Hyattsville, Md.: U.S. Department of Health and Human Services, Centers for Disease Control and Prevention, National Center for Health Statistics.

Mayberry, Robert, Fatima Mili, and Elizabeth Ofili. 2000. "Racial and Ethnic Differences in Access to Medical Care." *Medical Care Research and Review* 57 (suppl. 1): 108–45.

Metropolitan Life Insurance Company. 1997a. *The MetLife Juggling Act Study: Balancing Caregiving with Work and the Cost Involved.* Westport, Conn.

———. 1997b. *The MetLife Study of Employer Costs for Working Caregivers.* Westport, Conn.

Waidman, Timothy, and Shruti Rajan. 2000. "Racial and Ethnic Disparities in Health Care Access and Utilization: An Examination of State Variation." *Medical Care Research and Review* 57 (suppl. 1): 55–84.

Wallace, Steven. 1990. "The No-Care Zone: Availability, Accessibility, and Acceptability in Community-Based Long-Term Care." *Gerontologist* 30 (2): 254–61.

Weinick, Robin, Samuel Zuvekas, and Joel Cohen. 2000. "Racial and Ethnic Differences in Access to and Use of Health Care Services, 1977 to 1996." *Medical Care Research and Review* 57 (suppl. 1): 36–54.

White-Means, Shelley. 2000. "Racial Patterns in Disabled Elderly Persons' Use of Medical Services." *Journal of Gerontology: Social Sciences* 53B (2): S76–S89.

White-Means, Shelley, and Michael Thornton. 1990a. "Ethnic Differences in the Production of Informal Home Health Care." *Gerontologist* 30 (6): 758–68.

———. 1990b. "Labor Market Choices and Home Health Care Provision among Employed Ethnic Caregivers." *Gerontologist* 30 (6): 769–75.

PART THREE

Prospects for Long-Term-Care Policymaking at State and Federal Levels

7

Perspective on the Politics of Long-Term Care

Judith Feder

THE TWO HEALTH-CARE battles of the 1990s—the health reform debate of 1993–94 and the budget debate of 1995—place the challenges and opportunities of long-term-care politics in stark relief. During the health reform debate, along with the transformation of the nation's health-care financing, the Clinton Health Security Act proposed a transformation in the financing of long-term care. The bill proposed a massive infusion of federal funds into home care—specifically, through grants to states to support assistance to the functionally impaired regardless of age or income. In addition, the bill proposed to significantly liberalize standards for nursing-home eligibility under Medicaid, allowing Medicaid beneficiaries greater asset and income protection. Despite the enormity of this initiative in fiscal and service terms, only a handful of experts and advocates even remember its existence in the health reform package. Indeed, it never received any serious political attention.

Now shift to the budget debate only a year later—specifically, that part of the budget debate surrounding the Republican legislation that would have transformed Medicaid from an entitlement to individuals to a block grant to states. Did long-term care receive serious political attention here? Absolutely. The block grant proposal's threat to Medicaid's long-term-care protections was perhaps the Democrats' most powerful weapon in defeating the entire Republican proposal.

The contrast could not be clearer. A proposal to improve long-term-care financing generated little if any political attention. A threat to existing long-term-care financing, on the other hand, aroused a powerful political movement. On offense, long-term care is a weak political issue; on defense, it is a powerhouse.

Dissatisfaction with the current long-term-care system is widespread. Its quality can be abysmal. It provides far more support for the institutions people

107

do not want to enter than for care at home, where most people would prefer to stay. Its financial burdens are catastrophic, and its caregiving burdens on families overwhelming. It leaves an estimated one in five impaired individuals living in the community with unmet needs, their health endangered and their quality of life demeaned. Addressing these problems—improving the long-term-care system—is not on the policy or political agenda, however. At the same time that the importance of public policy to the existing long-term-care system is easily recognized (witness the 1995 budget debate), the importance of public policy to improving long-term-care financing is virtually ignored.

The challenge in long-term-care politics is to mobilize the issue's defensive power for purposes of offense—to generate the same political energy to advance the system as apparently exists to protect it. What will make that happen?

First, people and policymakers have to recognize that the way we currently deal with the risk of needing long-term care is not the only way to deal with it. The risk of needing long-term care can be spread through insurance, just as the risks of needing health care or disability or retirement income are spread. In popular discussion and public debate, the risk of needing long-term care is too often characterized both as an inevitable accompaniment to aging and as personally manageable. In fact, it is neither. We clearly need an insurance system to spread the risk of this unpredictable and unmanageable event.

Second, people and policymakers have to recognize that it will take a public policy initiative to put insurance coverage in place. Government does not have to provide all of that insurance. We can look for ways to promote public and private insurance to spread risk across taxpayers and individuals. The advancement of any successful insurance system, however, will require policy changes and public resources. In my view, priority in the use of public or taxpayer resources should be given to low- and modest-income people, for whom private resources are limited.

Third, an effective policy offensive will require confidence in government. That confidence depends on government's demonstrated ability to perform its current responsibilities in long-term care and other areas well. The horrific events of September 11, 2001, seem to have been followed by an upsurge of public confidence in government. We may have learned from that experience, as someone has noted, that "government is the enemy until you need a friend." People who need long-term care clearly need a friend. To be that friend, government has to work.

That leads to a fourth point—the need for oversight and advocacy to hold government accountable. The continuing challenge to ensure quality in nursing homes reveals the importance of oversight. Despite enactment of quality standards for nursing homes fifteen years ago, it is clear that without oversight by the U.S. General Accounting Office, performance of abysmal quality would remain invisible and unaddressed. Moreover, we can observe the power of advocacy in the effectiveness of the nonelderly disabled community in changing attitudes and policy toward disability. Despite the conventional wisdom about the political power of the elderly population, the bulk of the Medicaid resources spent on home- and community-based care are devoted to the younger, not the older, population with disabilities. Effective advocacy for the older population may require mobilization of their children. Indeed, the power of the baby-boom generation may first be evident in their advocacy for aging parents, well before they themselves have long-term-care needs.

Last but not least, an effective policy offensive will require money and leadership—more specifically, federal money and leadership. States shape and manage our current long-term-care system, with significant help from federal dollars. The current recession, however, has revealed the fragility of the system. States are struggling with fewer resources and higher costs, and support for long-term care is not immune from spending cuts. Furthermore, as long as we rely on state choices and state financing to determine long-term-care policies, protections will never be even or equitable across states, and protections in some states will be grossly inadequate. These inequities and inadequacies will only get worse as the population ages. Sooner rather than later, one hopes, the need for a national financing policy will become apparent.

None of these "necessary ingredients" for an effective offensive on long-term-care policy can be assumed to exist, though experience with an effective defense of long-term-care policy suggests that the power is there. The challenge is to mobilize it.

8

The View from the Office of the Assistant Secretary for Planning and Evaluation

Ruth Katz

A S THE PRINCIPAL ADVISER on policy development to the Secretary of the Department of Health and Human Services (HHS), the Office of the Assistant Secretary for Planning and Evaluation (ASPE) is responsible for major activities in the areas of policy coordination, legislation development, strategic planning, policy research and evaluation, and economic analysis. Our group, the Office of Disability, Aging, and Long-Term Care Policy, is charged with developing, analyzing, evaluating, and coordinating HHS and related policies and programs that support the independence, productivity, health, and long-term-care needs of people with disabilities, including children, working-age adults, and the elderly.

The current administration has a deep commitment to understanding the details and implications of the demographic changes we face as the population ages. We are living longer and are healthier than ever before, and aging baby boomers will have a major effect on the number of older people in the near future. The ASPE is interested in the implications of the graying of the population in terms of healthy aging and in terms of increased demand for long-term care. I commend the National Academy of Social Insurance and those who participated in its 2002 conference for taking a closer look at this important issue. As we all know, it is not going to go away—and we are all best served by a deeper understanding of the issues and an examination of possible solutions.

Another important message I bring is that the administration, and particularly Secretary of Health and Human Services Tommy Thompson, recognizes that this increased demand for long-term care presents a number of challenges and opportunities for the country. The federal government needs to work with states, with providers, with long-term-care consumers and their families. No solution to long-term-care issues will be found if the parties are polarized. There must be a partnership of private providers, consumers, states, and the federal government. All parties must do their part, even as we try to figure out what our respective roles should be.

The role of the federal government is frequently to get out of the way, and we should recognize when it is appropriate to do that. Medicaid, the principal payer of publicly funded long-term care, is a partnership, of course. However, many committed providers, individuals, and states are anxious to design innovative creative initiatives of their own; and one of the most effective moves that the federal government can do is get out of the way of these efforts. We recognize our role, but it is important to do as much as possible to allow innovation and creativity.

One of the long-standing primary goals of our office is to think broadly about long-term care: the range of services and the types of approaches available to elderly and disabled individuals and to informal caregivers. More recently we have also focused on giving people more choice and control over the services they receive so that their quality of life can be maintained and even improved. This is an agenda that should appeal to everyone.

Our office is looking for alternatives that are both consumer directed and market driven. Through our three state Cash and Counseling Demonstrations, we have learned that when people get more choice and control over their own services, they have better health outcomes, they use fewer nursing-home services, they stay home longer, they are happier, they are in control of their own lives. The success of the cash-and-counseling programs is stunning; the satisfaction rate has been 99 percent.

We are working aggressively with our partners inside the Department of Health and Human Services, the Centers for Medicare and Medicaid Services, and elsewhere to find other ways to enable states to offer consumer direction as "business as usual" rather than as a special demonstration waiver. We would like to see it become part of the normal way that states offer services. CMS recently published the "Independence Plus" waiver templates to make it easier for states to apply for waivers to offer consumer-directed programs.

We can also be of some help with respect to the worker shortage in the long-term-care industry. To date, the ASPE has focused most of its energy in long-term care on the direct-care work force. We cannot, of course, simply provide more direct-care workers and registered nurses to deliver services. Long-term care is not always a first choice for people in the market for minimum-wage jobs. It is a demanding job, both physically and mentally. We need to find ways to improve the dignity of direct-care workers and to improve management, to ease some of the burdens of their jobs. Some early findings show that it is quite possible to make some changes through management approaches, creation of career ladders, and other practices.

The Administration on Aging's National Family Caregiver Support Program has generated a great deal of enthusiasm within the present administration, in the states, and among consumers, researchers, and family members. Most long-term care is provided free of charge, informally by family members and friends, and the Caregiver Support Program was designed to support those caregivers. While I was working with the Long-Term Care Work Group during health care reform, informal caregivers often reminded us that they were not looking to pass responsibilities for aging parents or disabled children on to someone else. They were committed to the care of their loved ones; but it is a heavy load to carry alone. If offered a huge package of comprehensive services, some caregivers would no doubt reject parts of that package. They just want a little bit of help and a little bit of relief, such as that provided by the Caregiver Support Program.

In the Olmstead Executive Order, President George W. Bush directed HHS and other agencies to identify and work to eliminate federal rules, regulations, and policies that impede the provision of home- and community-based services to people with disabilities. Certainly some of the more obvious impediments are to be found in some of the rules in the Medicaid program.

"Delivering on the Promise," an HHS report issued at the end of 2001, includes more than twenty proposals for the ASPE.[1] We have already begun to implement some of them; others will require development of legislative proposals and will take a little longer. Still others will probably be part of the 2003 budget.

The complaint is often heard that federal programs are inconsistent across the government. Secretary Thompson has made a commitment to working closely with other federal agencies to address inconsistencies and thereby to better serve consumers. We have often organized discussions among committed people from different departments who do not seem to speak the same language. I know this happens on a state and local level, as well. It is important that we recognize that we are all working toward the same goals and learn to communicate effectively with one another. Some of this requires greater flexibility for states so that the rules of one department do not bump into those of another: for example, differences in department eligibility rules might make a person eligible for an HHS program but ineligible for a similar program originating in the Department of Housing and Urban Development.

The Bush administration does not consider its role in promoting a wide range of long-term-care support services as limited to Medicare and Medicaid. The Centers for Medicare and Medicaid Services, for instance, is getting ready

1. U.S. Department of Health and Human Services (2001).

to test a long-term-care awareness campaign to encourage seniors and those planning their retirement to think about the risk of needing long-term care and to incorporate long-term-care planning into their retirement planning.

The need to plan for possible long-term-care needs seems obvious to some providers and policymakers, who think about long-term care for a living, but for most people it is far from intuitive. Like many of the conference participants, I work in a long-term-care office. My office is within a larger policy office, and I am often approached by a colleague with a personal question: "Something just happened to my mother, and we need long-term care. What can we do"? I am proud to say that we have a knowledgeable staff—though we are not caseworkers, we are policy analysts—who usually provide the assistance sought. The questioner's first thought is usually, "What do I do to get Medicare to pay for this?" The answer, as often as not, is, "Medicare doesn't pay for that."

Recently, though, I experienced a new take on the whole question. A young woman who works down the hall in another office stopped by to see me because she had heard that our office is the long-term-care office. She said, gravely and earnestly, "I have a terrible problem. I just don't know what I'm going to do. I just got married and I just found out my husband's parents don't have long-term-care insurance." So it appears that at least one twenty-something in America is thinking about long-term-care insurance. Jokingly, I thought of a great advertising campaign, too. "Your husband's parents don't have long-term care insurance? Why didn't you work that out before you married the guy?"

The point of the long-term-care planning campaign of the Centers for Medicare and Medicaid Services is to get more people thinking like that—not scared and troubled about it, simply thinking about it as a step in long-term planning, similar to selecting a health insurance plan. As much as we might dislike thinking about ourselves as eventual users of long-term care, we must still be prepared for that possibility. I think Secretary Thompson's interest in this is simply to give people some idea of the options available and to suggest that they inform themselves about which services Medicare does and does not cover.

Private insurance, of course, is one answer for some people, and the Bush administration is interested in making it easier for people who want to plan ahead in this way to be able to do so. The president has endorsed a tax deduction for the purchase of long-term-care insurance policies, and we are actively looking at other measures to make long-term-care insurance more available.

Our office sponsored the first study ever conducted that surveyed the experiences of private long-term-care insurance policyholders who had triggered their benefits and were using them to purchase long-term-care services. The study finds, once again, that people want flexibility, the same flexibility we are working on in the Medicaid program, to give people more choices, more control. Those are the kinds of long-term-care insurance policies that people want to have, offering them options that include home care, bringing in the services needed to support their family members.

In evaluating the assessment instruments used in postacute care, we found that we were laboring under a bit of a misunderstanding: we had assumed that primary- and acute-health-care systems have good record-keeping and that communication between providers is adequate. We have learned, however, that that is not really the case; a number of inconsistencies exist across instruments.

In response, John Hoff, the deputy assistant secretary for disability, aging, and long-term care policy in the ASPE, has taken on as a leadership issue the vision of an electronic health-care record that spans acute, primary, and long-term care, into which providers can enter information once and use it many times. We are currently exploring ways to achieve that vision. It is a long-range vision, not one that will materialize in a year or two. However, we can start to imagine how we might use the advantages of the information age to improve the delivery of health-care services. Electronic records could mean that consumers would not have to keep repeating information and that providers would have all the information they need at their fingertips. This idea comes out of a strong commitment, shared by Deputy Assistant Secretary Hoff and Secretary Thompson, to consumer-directed health and long-term-care systems.

Reference

U.S. Department of Health and Human Services. 2001. *Delivering on the Promise: Compilation of Individual Federal Agency Reports of Actions to Eliminate Barriers and Promote Community Integration.* Report to the President on Executive Order 13217. Compiled by the U.S. Department of Health and Human Services, New Freedom Initiative Work Group, led by the Centers for Medicare and Medicaid Services and the Office for Civil Rights.

9

The Role of States in Long-Term-Care Reform

Joshua M. Wiener

W HAT ROLE SHOULD THE states play in long-term-care reform, and what are the likely consequences of depending on the states as the focal point of innovation? Long-term care is a large component of state health policy and state funding for health care. In 1998 long-term care represented 42 percent of Medicaid expenditures (excluding administration and disproportionate-share hospital payments) and 14 percent of all state and local health-care spending.[1] About half of these Medicaid expenditures were for the elderly population. Because of the high cost of long-term-care services (in 2000 a year in a nursing home cost an average of $49,000), Medicaid coverage for long-term care provides a safety net for the middle class as well as the poor.[2]

Although the federal government finances much of long-term care through Medicaid, the states dominate long-term-care policy. States set Medicaid and other public program reimbursement rates, control supply through certificate-of-need programs and moratoriums on new construction, decide what to cover through their own programs and through Medicaid, and assess clients and determine what services they will receive.

State control of the policy levers is consistent with the fact that long-term care is local and personal. Long-term care is idiosyncratic and directly relates to how we live our lives. Arguably, states are better able than the federal government to respond to local preferences and norms. Indeed, in many countries, local or at least subnational entities and organizations play a major role in the financing and delivery of services.[3]

---

1. Bruen and Holahan (2001); Centers for Medicare and Medicaid Services, *National Health Expenditures, by Source of Funds and Type of Expenditures, Calendar 1994–1999* (www.cms.hhs.gov/statistics/nhe/historical/t3.asp [September 26, 2002]).

2. Office of National Health Statistics (2002); Wiener, Sullivan, and Skaggs (1996).

3. Wiener (1996).

Service Delivery

In evaluating the potential role of states in reform, one prime factor is past performance: what have states already done with their flexibility and responsibility in this area? State innovation has been strongest in the area of service delivery. In virtually all states, a major policy priority is creation of a more balanced delivery system, with more emphasis on home- and community-based services. Despite this goal, however, the reality is that the vast majority of Medicaid funds are still spent on institutional care rather than for home- and community-based services. In 1998 only about 16 percent of Medicaid long-term-care expenditures for the older population went toward provision of home- and community-based services.[4]

Although state-funded programs are important in filling the gaps and providing services to persons who do not qualify for Medicaid, most funding for home care is provided through Medicaid. In most states, the attraction of the federal dollars available with Medicaid funding has eclipsed state-funded programs. Within Medicaid, states are increasingly relying on waivers for home- and community-based services to fund these services.

Medicaid home- and community-based services waivers allow states to develop innovative and flexible benefit packages that meet the needs of people with disabilities and give states mechanisms to control spending that are otherwise absent from the Medicaid program. Federal requirements mean that waivers operate more like appropriated programs than open-ended entitlements. In particular, states may establish waiting lists for waiver services, something that is not permitted in the normal Medicaid program. This lack of entitlement takes away state fears that unmet need for services (the "woodwork effect") will result in a large increase in demand and expenditures. Thus, under the waivers, states need not fear an explosion in expenditures.

The states have pursued two main innovations in home- and community-based services. The first is consumer-directed home care, under which individual consumers rather than agencies do the hiring, training, scheduling, and firing of the workers. The second is the use of nonmedical residential settings, such as assisted-living residences and adult family homes—facilities that are able to obtain the economies of scale of institutions like nursing homes but with a more homelike environment and without the medical model. Both strategies are designed to increase consumer autonomy and to cost less than other ways of providing care.

4. Urban Institute analysis of Health Care Financing Administration Forms 64 and 2082, available from the author.

Financing

States have been less innovative in terms of financing. Eighteen states offer a tax deduction or credit for purchase of private long-term-care insurance, but the incentives are probably too small to induce many people to purchase policies.[5] In addition, four states have instituted a public-private partnership, under which people who purchase a state-approved private long-term-care insurance policy can keep more of their assets and still qualify for Medicaid long-term-care benefits. Few people have purchased these policies, however, despite a substantial effort to promote them. No state has adopted a social insurance program for long-term care, although Hawaii has considered it.

States have done a little in terms of capitation and integration of services. In terms of integration of acute- and long-term-care services provided through managed-care organizations, there has been a lot of talk but not much has happened. Blending Medicare and Medicaid has proved to be difficult, partly because of the different philosophies of the two programs regarding mandatory enrollment in managed care and partly because of federal concerns about what will happen to the Medicare money in these capitated arrangements. Minnesota, Arizona, and Texas have some initiatives to integrate acute- and long-term-care services, but these demonstrations address only Medicaid-funded services. Michigan and Wisconsin have experimented with capitation and integration of long-term-care services only.

Especially given the current fiscal pressures, states are spending a lot of their energy and creativity on finding ways to maximize federal Medicaid dollars. In the past, they have focused on shifting expenditures for home health care and skilled-nursing facilities from Medicaid to Medicare. More recently, public nursing homes are heavily involved in a variety of so-called upper-payment-limit schemes designed to increase federal Medicaid payments without the need for states to spend any additional money.[6]

Quality Assurance

The federal government overwhelmingly dominates quality assurance for nursing homes. Indeed, fears about what would happen if states were solely responsible for both the financing and the quality assurance of nursing homes was a major reason for the political failure of the proposed Medicaid block grant in 1995 and 1996.

5. Wiener, Tilly, and Goldenson (2000).
6. Holahan, Wiener, and Lutzky (2002).

On the other hand, states do control the quality assurance process for home care. A fair assessment is that though they have done some things to ensure quality, the level of effort has been modest. States have focused instead on expanding services. The basic premise of the move toward home- and community-based services has been that the quality would be better than in nursing homes, but there are few data with which to evaluate that claim one way or the other.

Conclusion

What does all of this imply about the wisdom of setting up the states as the engine of long-term-care reform? First, long-term care is clearly higher on the political agenda of states than on that of the federal government. This is because of the relative fiscal importance of long-term care to the states, as well as the fact that they have more day-to-day responsibility for operating the system. As the population ages, both factors may change at the federal level, but that is not likely to occur for some time.

Second, as in every area in which states have flexibility, there is great variation in state activity. Some states are innovative, but many are not. Some states spend a lot on home- and community-based services, and others do not. Wherever there is that kind of variation, the issue of horizontal equity must be acknowledged. People with similar income and assets, levels of disability, and informal care supports but living in different states receive different publicly funded services. It is hard to rationalize those differences, and a part of the traditional role of the federal government has been to lessen those variations.

Third, states have been innovative in terms of service delivery (especially using Medicaid home- and community-based services waivers), but they have done little in terms of financing or quality assurance for home care. No state has tried to move dramatically toward either private or social insurance; all have stayed within the structures given them by the federal government in terms of the Medicaid program.

Regarding service delivery, much of long-term care is personal and local. From that perspective, Medicare may not be the proper vehicle to foster the kinds of innovations desired in provision of services. Medicare is a uniform national program and is likely to be too rigid and too bureaucratic to be the optimal vehicle for delivery of those services. However, non-means-tested financing—which is desirable—is not dependent on using Medicare to finance long-term care.

Finally, given the current political environment, incremental reforms may be all that is feasible at this time. The State Children's Health Insurance

Program (SCHIP) could provide a model of how the states and the federal government can work together to change the long-term-care system, especially in terms of home- and community-based services. The program has been politically popular and quite successful in providing health insurance to children from modest-income households that are ineligible for Medicaid. The program has been successful for three reasons: First, the federal government provides high matching rates; a great deal of federal money, and relatively little state money goes into SCHIP coffers. Financially, states have been given "an offer they couldn't refuse." Second, states have considerable flexibility in how they meet the goal of insuring children. This has given them a strong sense of ownership of the program, even though their financial contribution has been modest. Third, states do not have to operate SCHIP as an entitlement program—a legal obligation to provide benefits regardless of its budget impact—which insulates them from the fear of runaway costs.

Long-term-care policy analysts with a long memory may recognize that these characteristics of SCHIP also applied to the long-term-care component of President Bill Clinton's health reform proposal of 1993 and 1994. Applying those program features—a high federal match, a great deal of state flexibility, and limited financial exposure—to a new long-term-care program for home- and community-based services could help change the balance of the delivery system, even out interstate disparities in coverage, and provide people with disabilities the services they need.

References

Bruen, Brian, and John Holahan. 2001. *Medicaid Spending Growth Remained Modest in 1998, but Likely Headed Upward.* Washington: Kaiser Family Foundation.

Holahan, John, Joshua M. Wiener, and Amy Westphahl Lutzky. 2002. "Health Policy for Low-Income People: State Responses to New Challenges." *Health Affairs, web exclusive,* May 22, 2002.

Office of National Health Statistics. 2002. "Estimated Spending for Freestanding Nursing Home Care, Calendar Years 1960–2000." Unpublished data. Baltimore: Centers for Medicare and Medicaid Services.

Wiener, Joshua M. 1996. "Long-Term Care Reform: An International Perspective." In *Health Care Reform: The Will to Change,* Health Policy Studies 8, 67–79. Paris: Organization for Economic Co-operation and Development.

Wiener, Joshua M., Catherine M. Sullivan, and Jason Skaggs. 1996. *Spending Down to Medicaid: New Data on the Role of Medicaid in Paying for Nursing Home Care.* Washington: AARP.

Wiener, Joshua M., Jane Tilly, and Susan M. Goldenson. 2000. "Federal and State Initiatives to Jump Start the Market for Private Long-Term Care Insurance." *Elder Law Journal* 8 (1): 57–102.

10

Long-Term-Care Policy in the New Reality

David Durenberger

T HERE IS A NEW political agenda in the United States since September 11, 2001, and although we cannot be sure how long it will last, it is important to discuss its impact on health and long-term-care issues. The previous agenda and the political dialogue around it were focused on issues like Social Security reform, Medicare reform, and at least $300 billion worth of prescription drugs. Discussion of immigration liberalization with the president of Mexico was a big issue three days before the September 11 attacks. Immigration issues are now focused instead on finding and exposing lapses and weaknesses in our immigration services. Stem-cell research and its funding, privacy protections, and education were also issues that would have been included in the political agenda of the next year or two. The primary issues on the new agenda are national security, homeland defense, bioterrorism, economic stimulus, energy, income protection, and what I call appropriations health care, according to which health-care policy is made by limiting the amount of money appropriated to important issues and reforms.

The president of the United States has an almost unprecedented 85 percent approval rating right now (January 2002). I imagine one of the things his father might tell him, reflecting on his own experience of similar situations, is, "Son, don't squander your political capital." So the big challenge for those of us who believe in bold thinking and for the people in leadership positions taking charge of the agenda is how to articulate our vision and how much of that political capital can or will be used over the next several years to achieve our goals.

Recently two public opinion pollsters, one Democrat and one Republican, using the same data, came to the same conclusion in their annual assessment of public opinion: the biggest issue in this country by far—twice as big as terrorism—is the economy. Interestingly, within the economy, the pollsters report that the number-one issue is health care.

Urgent versus Important Issues

What are the primary issues of long-term care? Politically, we need to distinguish between the urgent issues and the important issues. One of the urgent concerns is the issue of reimbursement, such as increased Medicaid matching rates. Medicaid cost increases, for which long-term-care costs are a primary driver, have pushed a significant number of states—somewhere between thirty and forty of them—into deficit right now, and the states are clamoring for relief. Staving off Medicare funding cuts is also an urgent issue, as is the work-force crisis, for the long-term-care industry. Both are critically important to ensuring quality care for the elderly. Until September 11 these issues could have been expected to appear on the next legislative agenda.

The important issues—those that are very much in need of change and important to the future of long-term care but not critical to the system's immediate functioning—have been buried even deeper on Washington's agenda. These issues include financing reform; systemic change; care directed by the consumer, not state government; housing as an element of long-term care; and long-term care as a basic component of financial security. All of these are still waiting on Washington for recognition and inclusion in the political dialogue.

Unless we begin to integrate the urgent and the important we will never fully develop a national dialogue or solution before the important becomes urgent. With a complicated issue like long-term care, which involves components of health and financial security, housing, family caregiving, and a constantly expanding continuum of care, we must take time to address the "important" so that we can truly enhance the economic and financial security of all Americans during times of need.

One Leader Cannot Do It All

Today, the urgent as well as the important issues are being addressed by only 1 of the 535 people who serve in Congress: John Breaux, the Democratic senator from Louisiana. Many people in Congress are talking about their concern for long-term care, but only Senator Breaux has focused on the important, not just the urgent. With so little real support in Congress, the issue could nonetheless reach the policy agenda if it had support in the White House. Unfortunately, right now, the immediate issues of national security are consuming the president and his staff. Furthermore, there is no overwhelming political ideology driving other issues in the absence of presidential initiative because we are perfectly divided politically right down the middle—not just in the Congress but in the state legislatures and the governorships, as well. The issues debate is not framed in a context of which party has the right answer because there is no debate.

To begin a debate and to convince more leaders of the importance of the issue, people in need of care, their families, and the men and women who provide their care and services must seek out and support candidates who are committed to addressing long-term-care issues. As our leaders themselves— and their parents—age, more of them will be having experiences with long-term care, and they need to recognize that their experiences are not unique but, rather, reflect the experience of millions of ordinary people. Only when we give adequate voice to the millions experiencing long-term care will we be able to engage in a national dialogue. Only when we can convince our most influential leaders of the growing need can we expect them to undertake reform.

Reform of the System

Too often in discussion of reform the focus is on controlling expenditures because of the absence of vision, leadership, and common agreement on where reform should be taking us. As a result, policy tends toward "incremental-ism"—an approach best expressed in the Yogi Berra saying, "If you don't know where you're going, any road will get you there." Policymakers resort to commissions and task forces, which, in the absence of an immediate crisis, have never produced an actionable vision for reform.

The problem with state reform, in this particular area, is that long-term care is a problem of financial and economic security. Long-term care is a national responsibility, and the states are not the best facilitators of financial and economic security. The governors of the states all think they govern more efficiently than Washington; and perhaps most states do. However, the finan-cial and health security of society's most vulnerable is not state specific.

After twenty-five years of state-specific reforms in the form of waivers and demonstrations, such as the On Lok program in California, which of the successful programs has been adopted on a national scale? If every state continues to operate on waivers and demonstration projects, the quality of care of disabled people will be determined by where they live. With a national policy that incorporates the success of these waived and demonstration pro-grams, states could devote their time to improving the efficiencies of the local service delivery systems—something they do best.

Another problem with treating this as a state reform problem is what I call the Minnesota "swing," a surplus-deficit problem. A year ago Minnesota, like many other states, had a significant budget surplus; today the state is $3 billion in debt, owing to a slowing economy and escalating costs. What is that going to mean for long-term-care financing? A state's financial capacity determines the quality of its long-term-care choices and consumers' access to services, because states finance those choices. With a national long-term-care financing reform effort, people in _____ them would not be subject to such immedia_____ issue here remains gove_____ making choices, becau_____ therefore make the dec_____ money flows to the indi_____ and the market respon_____

Why the Delay in

Why the delay in _____ at commands attention _____ a significant number o_____ it. Long-term care is _____ ble decline that ends onl_____ t to address. This public _____ out the value of independ_____ king about the aging side of disability—from the developmental_____ and their families, who utilize tremendous amounts of long-term care.

Ultimately, long-term-care reform has been unable to get the attention it deserves because it lacks a strong "wedge"—an issue to which it can be attached to drive it into the public and political consciousness. Long-term care needs a wedge, a significantly large and politically salient issue that involves many of the same health and financial security issues that make up long-term-care financing. Entitlement reform in the form of Social Security and Medicare could serve as such a wedge in the long-term-care debate. In the 1930s, when financial security was challenged, and in the 1960s, when it was challenged again, we turned to national social insurance programs to help support economic security. We need to turn there again today, not to create a new program but to take programs created in the 1930s and the 1960s and adapt them to work for us in the twenty-first century. The initiative should make policymakers recognize the threat that inadequate planning for long-term care represents to health and financial security.

Another wedge might be the uninsured. Ninety-four percent of all Americans are without long-term-care insurance. Long-term care is an insurable event, but the insurance industry will not offer a truly affordable private long-term-care insurance product until the Social Security Administration and the Centers for Medicare and Medicaid Services decide how they are going to treat long-term care.

In sum, we need a national dialogue that connects long-term care to financial security. It must be led by the president of the United States and everybody else who is in what we call the power structure in America. The power structure must address the need for long-term care and health care as potential threats to the financial security of every American and, therefore, to the economic security of our country. I am reminded of the words of Winston Churchill, "Americans always do what's right, but only after they've tried everything else." We have tried everything else; it is now time to address long-term-care reform as it rightly is: a key component of the financial security of every American and therefore a national security issue deserving of national attention.

Commentary on Part Three

Comment by John Rother

I am a son of a preacher, and so I know when I have been invited to preach to the choir. One of my frustrations, having worked in this field for so long, is that we have been talking solely to one another for too long and thus have missed some opportunities for improving long-term care in this country. Therefore, I would like to discuss ways we can make better use of the opportunities that will come again in long-term care. From a grassroots point of view, one might think that this issue would provoke a lot of political activism. Judy Feder is quite right to say that, though we have tried, the results are disappointing. There are some important reasons, however, for the issue's failure to ignite in the past; and the first is that this is a scary subject, especially in these United States of Denial.

For people who are already elderly, long-term care is too scary to discuss. The most common response I get when trying to initiate conversation about long-term care with people in their seventies or eighties is, "I would rather die than be a burden to my children, be dependent, lose control over my life, or go to a nursing home. I don't want to talk about it." The message might be better received if we talked instead to their children—the baby boomers.

The second obstacle is that we have been talking about nursing homes way too much. A nursing home is not a place anyone wants to go. My mother right now is in a very good one, but she is anxious to get out of it. Senator David Durenberger hits the nail on the head: long-term care tied to nursing homes is not an issue that resonates with the American people. We should be talking instead about independent living. We should be talking about what people want rather than what they fear.

Third, the population in general is uninformed on the issue. AARP conducted a telephone poll in December 2001 in which more than 30 percent of the

125

adults over the age of 45 who responded assured us that they were already covered for long-term care. It will be hard to sell a new policy initiative if a large part of the public thinks they are already protected.

So what are we doing to do about it? Well, AARP is planning to launch a major initiative in 2002 to address the full continuum of needs, from independent living through long-term care to the end of life. It is going to be an ambitious multiyear effort focused on education and information. It will push hard to expand home- and community-based options. It will address quality and, ultimately, financing. We at AARP will try to break through some of this denial and some of this ignorance, but we do not plan to do it on our own. We are looking for partners, hoping to team up with many other organizations.

In addition to this campaign, a fresh approach to public policy would be a productive reform. Long-term-care reform may prove a more palatable topic if it is broken down into five dimensions. The first should be family caregiving, because that is what the baby-boom generation is currently facing. In this regard, AARP has a proposal on the table, sponsored by Senators Bob Graham and Chuck Grassley and Representatives Nancy Johnson and Karen Thurman, that would provide a $3,000 tax credit to family caregivers. This tax credit alone is not going to solve the problem, but it is a beginning. I think we can get this passed into law, if not this year, in the next few years.

Second, we could continue to build on the great work that On Lok started in terms of integration of services, especially for the dually eligible. The money is there. It is capitated, so we can be creative about how we use it. Third, the political interest in Medicare reform gives us an opportunity to think about how to change Medicare to make it a more appropriate program for dealing with chronic illness and disability. Fourth, when it comes to services, baby boomers like choice and control—consumer-directed care. Consumer-based models of care offer much promise. Disability models, not medical models, are more appealing to consumers. Finally, housing is too often a neglected part of long-term care. We have to think not only about what housing we build but also, and even more important, about how aging proceeds in existing retirement communities: how can services be provided there to keep people from being forced into institutions?

In sum, if long-term-care issues can be broken down into their constituent parts, maybe the topic can be made easier to digest. If we change the language, maybe it can be made more politically appealing. If we talk to the baby boomers, maybe it can be made less scary. In the end, we can start to make some progress on this issue only if we work together on the different elements and talk about long-term care in a new way.

Comment by Joanne Silberner

The preceding chapters have presented a number of interesting ideas, interesting thoughts, and interesting possibilities. Why do we not hear them from the media?

As journalists, we in the media try either to find news or to find stories. Sometimes we find both. Stories have narrative, and they are more often heard on National Public Radio (NPR) than on other radio and television networks, more often in magazine articles than in the Associated Press or in the *Washington Post* or the *New York Times*. In narratives, something happens; something changes. For example, new federal or state programs may generate a narrative story. Joe Shapiro reported a story for NPR a while ago on a New Hampshire waiver that allows lump sums of money to go to Medicaid recipients. The story focused on two sisters; one was disabled, the other was caring for her. It was a great story because as listeners learned about the waiver program they also learned about the sisters.

I did a piece on dedicated parents who were losing custody of their child because he needed full-time care; the State of Virginia's Medicaid program did not support full-time care at home and would not make an exception in his case. The parents signed over custody to the state so that their child could receive the care he needed, but they lost their child. That's a story. Something happens. There are people involved, and something changes.

News is also something happening, but endless debate does not count. Media can cover the introduction of a new idea, such as legislation that is actually moving forward. Media cannot cover legislation being introduced just to sit there. Media will not cover another commission.

It is hard to interest our listeners and readers in long-term-care issues because they have seen it all before. For the media to discuss long-term care, something has to be changing. We will cover a new program. We will cover the beginning and the ending of a program, but we do not cover the middle—the everyday stories—so well.

Paul Kleyman, the editor of *Aging Today,* is quite passionate about issues of aging and long-term care. He once complained to me that "the zookeepers in politics keep shouting that we have to worry about the pachyderm Medicare before we cover long-term care." The editors at NPR concur. Medicare is a topic that we can cover because it is an issue with clear political agendas. Long-term care, however, is more muddied, and it is not a pachyderm. So the media covers a budget fight, policy changes, bankruptcies, and scandals involving long-term care.

Radio requires sound, and television visuals. Thanks to the baby boomers, sex, drugs, and music are also part of the package. Long-term care does not often offer these components. Baby boomers are the reporters and the editors right now, and baby boomers do not much want to think about long-term care. It is the ostrich syndrome. Baby boomers cannot remember life without Medicare or Social Security. These programs have always been there, so we assume that long-term care will be there when we need it. This is the assumption of the generation of people who are making news decisions now—something will come along.

Moreover, not many reporters, at least in Washington, are covering aging issues. Paul Kleyman puts the number at fewer than ten. Even fewer cover disability issues full-time. In contrast with major media, the trade press is doing a good job covering age and disability issues.

The good news is that NPR is committed to covering issues of long-term care and especially issues of the disabled; Paul Kleyman has noted that the Knight Center for Specialized Journalism has a special course in this. At the upcoming meeting of the Association of Health Care Journalists, of which I am a board member, there will be a special session on aging.

Ultimately, news is something that happens to editors. So though the past may be grim, in terms of news coverage of long-term care, I expect it to change—not, perhaps, for the right reasons, but it is going to change.

PART FOUR

Building on Experience: What Have We Learned about Meeting Needs for Chronic and Long-Term Care?

11

Ensuring Quality in Long-Term-Care Settings

Catherine Hawes

THE "GRAYING" OF America represents a major challenge to individuals, to families, and to our society. Our success in treating acute illness and extending the life span of Americans has led to the rapid growth of the population aged 65 and older, many of whom suffer from chronic diseases. Some of these individuals will need long-term care to help them deal with the limitations in physical or cognitive function associated with chronic disease.

The vast majority of persons needing long-term care will receive such help at home, from family members. However, more than two-fifths (43 percent) of all persons who turned 65 in 1990 or later will enter a nursing home at some time before they die.[1] The probability of use increases dramatically with age, rising from 17 percent for those 65 to 74 years of age to 60 percent for persons aged 85 to 94, the fastest growing segment of the population.

Many observers have focused on the need for private and public sector responses to meet this growing need for various types of long-term-care services.[2] Others have concentrated on the fiscal impact of these demographic and morbidity trends.[3] However, the issue of how to ensure quality of care for persons needing long-term care, particularly those who are the most impaired and will need the total care provided in a residential long-term-care setting, is an equally compelling issue.

Regulation Can Improve Quality

In some circles, regulation is not popular, particularly in this era of reliance on supposed market-based reforms and incentives for quality improvement.

1. Kemper and Murtaugh (1991); Murtaugh, Kemper, and Spillman (1990).
2. Williams and Temkin-Greener (1996).
3. Callahan (1987).

Despite its waning political popularity, however, regulation can improve quality, as shown in a variety of recent studies. One study, funded by the Office of the Assistant Secretary for Planning and Evaluation of the U.S. Department of Health and Human Services, examined the effect of regulation on the quality of care in board-and-care homes. This study ranked the regulatory systems in all fifty states based on their standards, inspection processes, and availability and use of enforcement remedies.[4] Five states with the most extensive regulatory systems and five with the most limited systems were then selected for study.

Analysis of primary data collected from a probability sample of residents, staff, and operators and observation of facilities reveals that quality was better along a number of dimensions in those states with more extensive regulatory systems.[5] States with more extensive regulatory systems were less likely to have unlicensed homes. In addition, facilities in such states were significantly less likely to be in the bottom quartile of board-and-care homes in a range of structural and process quality measures; thus more extensive regulatory systems were successful in minimizing the worst performance. Finally, quality was significantly better in board-and-care homes in states with more extensive regulatory systems in terms of a number of indicators of quality, including operator training, staff knowledge of the ombudsman program, availability of social and recreational aides, resident involvement in activities, rates of psychotropic drug use, rates of inappropriate medication use, and, interacting with the effect of licensure status, safety and the availability of key services and supportive devices. Moreover, these results were obtained without the negative effect feared by some—namely, that regulation would create a more "institutional," less homelike, environment.[6]

Several studies of nursing homes have also demonstrated the positive effect of regulation. For example, after the passage of the Omnibus Budget Reconciliation Act (OBRA) of 1987, a number of studies found a positive effect of OBRA on various aspects of process quality, including reductions in such negative practices as the use of physical restraints, the inappropriate use of psychotropic drugs, and the use of indwelling catheters.[7] Other studies have found increases in good care practices during the post-OBRA period, such as more accurate medical record-keeping, more comprehensive care plans, in-

4. Hawes, Mor, and others (1995).

5. Hawes, Mor, and others (1995); Wildfire and others (1997–98).

6. Hawes, Mor, and others (1995); Wildfire and others (1997–98).

7. Garrard, Chen, and Dowd (1995); Hawes and others (1997); Kane and others (1993).

creased presence of advanced directives, greater use of toileting programs for residents with bowel incontinence, and greater resident participation in activities.[8] In addition, reduced rates of decline in physical functioning, cognitive functioning, and urinary continence were observed, and there was a significant reduction in hospital use by nursing-home residents, with no increase in mortality.[9]

The 1987 OBRA also mandated use of the principles of geriatric assessment to improve the care of residents and to maximize their functioning. This was particularly critical because the average nursing-home resident has four chronic diseases that must be managed appropriately.[10] One of the chief features of the OBRA legislation was a new requirement that Medicare- and Medicaid-certified nursing facilities use a standardized, "reproducible," comprehensive functional assessment tool to evaluate all residents and guide the development of individualized care plans. This tool, known as the Resident Assessment Instrument (RAI), was developed under contract with the Centers for Medicare and Medicaid Services (formerly the Health Care Financing Administration).

The RAI consists of two parts. The Minimum Data Set for Nursing Home Resident Assessment and Care Screening (MDS) is the core functional assessment instrument in the RAI and covers such domains as physical functioning in the activities of daily living, cognition, continence, mood, behaviors, nutritional status, vision and communication, activities, and psychosocial well-being.[11] The purpose of the MDS assessment is to identify a resident's strengths, preferences, and needs in key areas and to provide a holistic and comprehensive picture of the resident's functional status. Each resident is assessed according to the MDS on admission and annually thereafter, as well as on any significant change in status. Residents are also assessed every three months, using a subset of MDS items.

The second part of the RAI comprises eighteen problem-focused Resident Assessment Protocols (RAPs) that specify additional, highly focused assessment to identify treatable causes of conditions that are common among nursing-home residents or that represent severe health risks. A RAP assessment is required if a resident's completed MDS suggests a problem, a risk for decline, or the potential for improved function in that area. These conditions, if present, trigger a resident for additional assessment that is specified under an explicit set of guidelines in each RAP. The focus of these guidelines is to help

8. Hawes and others (1997); Marek and others (1996); Teno and others (1997).
9. Phillips and others (1997); Mor and others (1997).
10. Strahan (1997).
11. Hawes, Morris, and others (1995); Morris and others (1990).

the facility identify and treat or manage chronic diseases, the onset of acute illnesses, adverse effects of medications, or other factors that caused or contributed to the functional problem or risk factor that triggered further clinical assessment. Thus the RAI is a critical element in managing chronic disease among residents and ensuring quality in long-term-care facilities.

Regulations That Encompass Accepted Clinical Practices Are Particularly Effective

Although the research demonstrated the effectiveness of the OBRA provisions early in their implementation, some of these studies also indicated that the areas in which there was the greatest impact were those in which the mandated practices were accepted by the provider community as clinically appropriate. For example, the two areas of greatest impact in the post-OBRA period were reductions in the use of physical restraints and the inappropriate use of psychotropic medications. Both had been the subject of considerable attention before the implementation of the OBRA regulations. The Health Care Financing Administration had convened clinical workgroups around the issue of the appropriate use of psychotropic medications in nursing homes. Indeed, there is evidence that this enhanced focus on reducing the inappropriate use of psychotropic medications and the increased attention to this issue among consulting pharmacists led facilities to initiate significant reductions in the use of psychotropic drugs after the passage of the OBRA legislation but before the date mandated for implementation of the regulations.[12]

The attention focused on reducing the use of physical restraints was even more significant. Consumer advocates had reported on practices in other countries that led to lower use of such devices. In addition, a group of nonprofit facilities in Pennsylvania, known as Kendall-Crossland, had nearly eliminated the use of physical restraints in their facilities and started a movement to "untie the elderly." Kendall-Crossland offered consultation to other facilities on how to reduce their use of physical restraints. This initiative did not lead to widespread reductions in other facilities across the nation, but it did help establish the OBRA mandate on the reduction of restraint use as a clinically important and achievable goal.

Facility-Based Interventions Can Also Improve Quality

As noted earlier in this paper, the OBRA mandates were fairly successful in reducing the use of physical restraints in nursing homes across the nation, with

12. Kane and others (1993).

Figure 11-1.   *Prevalence of Restraint Use, 1991 and 1993*

Percent

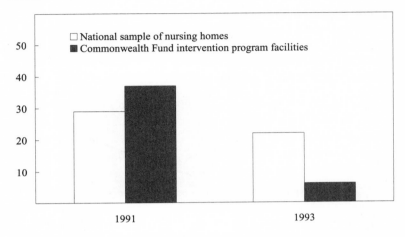

Source: Author's calculations based on federal survey data from Phillips, Wildfire, and Hawes (1998).

a drop from a pre-OBRA 1990 prevalence of nearly 40 percent to about 20 percent by 1994.[13] By 2000 the level of use had declined to between 13 and 14 percent,[14] although some facilities have achieved a much lower rate.

Clinical intervention and consultation, such as that embodied in the Commonwealth Fund's National Nursing Home Restraint Minimization Program in the early to middle 1990s, helped some facilities reduce their use of restraints. In the sixteen facilities enrolled in the intervention program, the prevalence of the use of restraints dropped to less than 5 percent. This intervention was extraordinarily successful in enabling facilities to go much further than they would have on their own, with only the impetus provided by regulatory incentives, as is illustrated in figure 11-1.

Unfortunately, once the Commonwealth Fund (CMWF) intervention ended, along with the fairly intensive consultation the CMWF had provided to the facilities, some of the nursing homes essentially abandoned what they had learned, for a variety of reasons—most notably, turnover in administrative

13. Hawes and others (1997); Kane and others (1993).

14. Personal communication from Charles D. Phillips based on analysis of data from the Online Survey and Confirmation Reports of the Health Care Financing Administration, Texas A&M University System Health Science Center, September 2000. See also Castle and Fogel (1998).

Figure 11-2.   *Prevalence of Restraint Use, 1991–96*

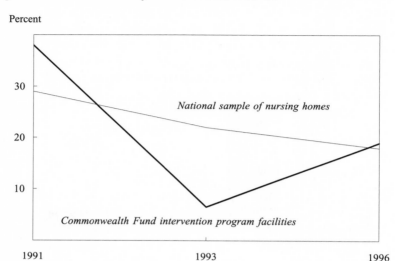

Percent

30

20

10

National sample of nursing homes

Commonwealth Fund intervention program facilities

1991   1993   1996

Source: Author's calculations based on federal survey data from Phillips, Wildfire, and Hawes (1998).

staff (for example, facility administrator and director of nursing). When follow-up data collection and analysis were conducted to examine restraint use in 1996, a disturbing pattern was observed. The result, aggregated across all the CMWF intervention facilities, is displayed in figure 11-2.

As this analysis demonstrates, the overall rate of restraint use in 1996 was essentially the same for the intervention nursing homes as for the nation. The average restraint use of the demonstration facilities in 1996 effectively rebounded to near the national norm from its much lower rate in 1993—a period at or near the end of the intervention. Most of the facilities maintained their much lower use; however, two facilities displayed a pattern of restraint use that was significantly higher than the national average rate.[15]

This failure among some of the sixteen facilities to maintain the low levels of restraint use illustrates the problem inherent in facility-based quality improvement initiatives: it is difficult to attain uniform implementation and to ensure persistence of the intervention over time. This phenomenon can also be seen in other interventions, from attempts to ensure that facilities follow best practices in the treatment and management of urinary incontinence to a broader intervention, such as the Wellspring Initiative.[16] The Wellspring Initiative,

15. Phillips, Wildfire, and Hawes (1998).
16. Personal communication from Jack Schnelle; Stone and others (2002).

originally introduced in eleven not-for-profit nursing homes in Wisconsin, has attained impressive results in reducing staff turnover among certified nurse assistants in participating facilities and in reducing the number of federal survey deficiencies in these nursing homes. Moreover, it has done so without increasing costs.[17] Yet an evaluation of the eleven original or "charter" facilities has found significant variation within and between facilities in their implementation of key aspects of the initiative. Moreover, this is true despite the fact that the facilities have maintained more than nominal commitment to participation in the Wellspring Initiative over a five-year period.

Good Quality Does Not Always Cost More

The facile assumption that improving quality always means increasing costs is clearly untrue. The actual relation between cost and quality is more complex, as noted by the Institute of Medicine in its seminal report, *Improving the Quality of Care in Nursing Homes*.[18] Indeed, consumer groups such as the National Citizens' Coalition for Nursing Home Reform have long argued, correctly, that there is a high cost of poor care, in both human and financial terms. More than that, some quality improvements have been achieved without increasing costs.

One of the first studies to examine the issue of the cost of a quality initiative in nursing homes focused on reducing the use of physical restraints. Some members of the nursing-home industry argued that implementing this provision of OBRA would increase nursing-home costs by more than $1 billion annually because more staff would be needed to deal with residents who had previously been restrained. However, empirical analysis of staff time studies indicates that residents who were restrained actually took more staff time than similar residents who were not restrained.[19]

An evaluation of the effect of OBRA and the implementation of the RAI also has found cost savings at the same time that quality improved. One study finds a significant reduction in hospital use among nursing-home residents.[20] This evaluation examined quality by collecting data on two independent cohorts of more than two thousand residents in a random sample of some 255 nursing facilities in ten states. If the results seen in these facilities had been obtained nationwide, that reduction in hospital use would have led to a

17. Stone and others (2002).
18. Institute of Medicine (1986).
19. Phillips, Hawes, and Fries (1993).
20. Mor and others (1997).

reduction in Medicare spending on inpatient acute care alone of more than $2 billion annually (in 1993 dollars).

Other studies have had similar results. The Wellspring Initiative, for example, was implemented with no total increase in costs to the participating facilities, although there was some reallocation of spending.[21] Two studies also examined nursing homes in New York and Ohio that attained higher-than-average quality and lower-than-expected costs.[22] These studies indicate that the nursing homes that succeeded did so using a variety of strategies and that the facilities differed in organizational structure and culture (for example, size, ownership, staff organization). What they shared was a "common commitment to quality and cost control."[23]

This finding—that some quality improvements can be obtained without an increase in costs—is important, particularly in times of fiscal constraint. That being said, it is equally important to note that some improvements cannot be achieved without increasing spending. The most notable example is staffing in nursing homes. To achieve a living wage for nursing assistants and to reach the staff-to-resident ratios many experts consider essential to quality nursing-home care, significant changes with substantial cost implications would be required. Indeed, in my view, this is the most essential change needed in the nation's nursing homes.

Ruminations on the Future: Lessons for Ensuring Quality in Long-Term Care

The long-term-care sector has both significant advantages and serious challenges. The advantages relate to what is known about how to ensure quality. First, long-term care now incorporates the best available evidence on effective practices in RAI and its RAPs. Second, it is more sophisticated than the acute- and ambulatory-care sectors in the development and use of quality indicators both for feedback to facilities and as a mechanism for targeting surveys.[24] Third, long-term care is more advanced than other health-care sectors in making uniform and up-to-date comparative information available to facilities through the Centers for Medicare and Medicaid Services' Nursing Home Compare website.[25]

21. Stone and others (2002).
22. Rudder and Phillips (1998); Phillips and Rose (2000).
23. Phillips (2002, p. 155).
24. Zimmerman (1998).
25. The Centers for Medicare and Medicaid Services website can be found at www.medicare.gov.

Long-term care can also benefit from the lessons about ensuring quality, including both the successes and limitations found in those studies. The difficulty of attaining uniform implementation of clinical interventions and of sustaining them over time suggests that efforts to improve and ensure quality in long-term-care facilities require more sophisticated approaches than are typical in long-term care; even regulatory mandates are not uniformly implemented across all facilities affected by the regulations.

Some evaluators of the Commonwealth Fund's restraint reduction initiative have concluded that the most successful strategy for reducing restraints combined the "push" of federal regulation with the "pull" generated by intensive, individualized consultation. In fact, this is an approach adopted to some degree by the Department of Social and Health Services in Washington state. Washington has long been regarded as having one of the most aggressive systems for regulating nursing homes.[26] Its nurse surveyors all have postgraduate degrees in nursing. The state has a strict policy of aggressively citing deficiencies and citing them at appropriate levels of scope and severity. Furthermore, Washington makes use of state remedies that it feels enable the survey agency to respond more quickly and effectively to deficiencies than it could with federal remedies, but it also uses a range of federal and state remedies appropriate to the nature of the deficiency and the history of the facility.[27]

In addition to having a proactive and aggressive regulatory approach, Washington state provides consultation to facilities that voluntarily participate in the Quality Assurance Nurse (QUAN) program. Approximately 80 percent of Washington's nursing homes choose to participate in the program. Until recently, they received consultation and training from the QUAN nurses, who are separate from the survey agency staff. The QUAN nurses provide education and training to facilities about the most up-to-date clinical practices and help them develop quality improvement initiatives, including steps to ensure effective implementation. In addition, they monitor the performance of the facilities and may visit as often as monthly to check on progress and work with the facility staff. During my recent interviews with key stakeholders about the nursing-home complaint investigation process, a variety of providers spontaneously praised the QUAN program and testified to the importance of this initiative in ensuring and improving quality in nursing homes. Finally, more than most states, Washington appears to have achieved a genuine partnership

26. Edelman (1998); Harrington, Mullan, and Carrillo (2001).
27. Edelman (1998); Harrington, Mullan, and Carrillo (2001); Hawes (2002).

among the nursing-home providers, consumers and their advocates, and the regulatory agency.[28]

This suggests that promising models of regulation and facility-sponsored initiatives exist. These warrant additional and more structured evaluation. We also need to determine the factors that account for differential performance across facilities—differences that are apparent in the implementation of both regulatory mandates and self-selected, facility-initiated quality improvement strategies. As Charles D. Phillips notes in a recent editorial in the *Gerontologist*, it is important to understand the impact of organizational structures, processes, and culture on facility performance;[29] however, it is equally important to examine the more amorphous attributes of a facility that affect its adoption and implementation of clinical initiatives and its compliance with state and federal regulations. Phillips characterizes these as the facility "leadership's commitment to quality and its openness to quality-related innovation."[30] Only as we come to understand and affect these factors can we ensure more uniform quality in nursing homes, whether through regulation or facility-based clinical interventions.

This effort to ensure quality cannot ignore the fact that there is substantial evidence of poor quality in many nursing homes and of failed regulatory processes.[31] Funding for nursing-home care waxes and wanes, as does the political will to enforce quality standards. Moreover, policymakers are often distracted by the search to avoid the fiscal implications of an aging society and the black hole that nursing-home expenditures represent for state and federal Medicaid budgets. Thus some chase after what they regard as easy panaceas, investing private long-term-care insurance and assisted living with mythical properties and giving them largely uncritical approbation. These factors distract us from the immediate and necessary challenge of ensuring that all nursing homes approach the level of quality demonstrated in the best facilities in the nation, of ensuring that all nursing homes reach the level of quality observed by resident Sallie Tisdale and reported in her article, "Harvest Moon: Portrait of a Nursing Home": "Ordinary, even familial things happen here, though often unwitnessed. Wounds are healed, muscles strengthened, faces washed, and hands held. Each small movement is tiny in its fruition, huge in its absence."[32]

28. Edelman (1998); Hawes (2002).

29. Phillips (2002, p. 156).

30. Phillips (2002, p. 155).

31. U.S. Department of Health and Human Services (1999a, 1999b); U.S. General Accounting Office (1998, 1999a, 1999b, 1999c, 2000); U.S. Senate (1997, 1998).

32. Tisdale (1987).

References

Callahan, Daniel. 1987. *Setting Limits: Medical Goals in an Aging Society*. Simon and Schuster.

Castle, Nick, and Barry Fogel. 1998. "Characteristics of Nursing Homes That Are Restraint Free." *Gerontologist* 38 (2): 181–88.

Edelman, Toby. 1998. "What Happened to Enforcement?" *Nursing Home Law Letter* (1–2): 1–46.

Garrard, Judy, V. Chen, and B. Dowd. 1995. "The Impact of the 1987 Federal Regulations on the Use of Psychotropic Drugs in Minnesota Nursing Homes." *American Journal of Public Health* 85 (6): 771–76.

Harrington, Charlene, Joe Mullan, and Helen Carrillo. 2001. *State Nursing Home Enforcement Systems*. Report prepared for the Kaiser Commission on Medicaid and the Uninsured. San Francisco: University of California, Department of Social and Behavioral Sciences.

Hawes, Catherine. 2002. *Assuring Quality in Nursing Homes: The Role of Enforcement*. Final report to the Retirement Research Foundation from the Program on Aging, Disability, and Long-Term Care Policy. College Station: Texas A&M System Health Science Center, School of Rural Public Health.

Hawes, Catherine, Vincent Mor, and others. 1995. *Executive Summary: Analysis of the Effect of Regulation on the Quality of Care in Board and Care*. Research Triangle Park, N.C.: Research Triangle Institute.

Hawes, Catherine, J. N. Morris, and others. 1995. "Reliability Estimates for the Minimum Data Set for Nursing Home Resident Assessment and Care Screening (MDS)." *Gerontologist* 35 (2): 172–78.

Hawes, Catherine, and others. 1997. "The Impact of OBRA-87 and the RAI on Indicators of Process Quality in Nursing Homes." *Journal of the American Geriatrics Society* 45 (8): 977–85.

Institute of Medicine. 1986. *Improving the Quality of Care in Nursing Homes*. Washington: National Academy of Sciences Press.

Kane, R. L., and others. 1993. "Restraining Restraints: Changes in a Standard of Care." *Annual Review of Public Health* 14: 545–84.

Kemper, Peter, and Christopher Murtaugh. 1991. "Lifetime Use of Nursing Home Care." *New England Journal of Medicine* 324 (9): 595–600.

Marek, K. D., and others. 1996. "OBRA '87: Has It Resulted in Positive Change in Nursing Homes?" *Journal of Gerontological Nursing* 22 (12): 32–40.

Mor, Vincent, and others. 1997. "Impact of the MDS on Changes in Nursing Home Discharge Rates and Destinations." *Journal of the American Geriatrics Society* 45 (8): 1002–10.

Morris, J. N., and others. 1990. "Designing the National Resident Assessment Instrument for Nursing Homes." *Gerontologist* 30 (3): 293–307.

Murtaugh, Christopher, Peter Kemper, and B. C. Spillman. 1990. "The Risk of Nursing Home Use in Later Life." *Medical Care* 28 (10): 952–62.

Phillips, C. D. 2002. "Guest Editorial: Yali's Question and the Study of Nursing Homes as Organizations." *Gerontologist* 42 (2): 154–56.

Phillips, C. D., Catherine Hawes, and B. E. Fries. 1993. "Reducing the Use of Physical Restraints in Nursing Homes: Will It Increase Costs?" *American Journal of Public Health* 83 (3): 342–48.

Phillips, C. D., and Miriam Rose. 2000. *Expense Control Strategies in Nursing Homes: Examples from Higher-Quality Facilities with Lower Operating Costs.* Beachwood, Ohio: Myers Research Institute.

Phillips, C. D., Judith Wildfire, and Catherine Hawes. 1998. "Reexamining the Effect on Restraint Use of the Commonwealth Fund's National Nursing Home Restraint Minimization Project." Working paper. Beachwood, Ohio: Myers Research Institute.

Phillips, C. D., and others. 1997. "The Impact of the RAI on ADLs, Continence, Communication, Cognition, and Psychosocial Well-being." *Journal of the American Geriatrics Society* 45 (8): 986–93.

Phillips, C. D., and others. 1998. *Ninety-One Ideas for Reducing Costs, Enhancing Revenue, and Maintaining Quality in Nursing Homes.* New York: Nursing Home Community Coalition of New York.

Strahan, G. W. 1997. "An Overview of Nursing Homes and Their Current Residents: Data from the 1995 National Nursing Home Survey." In *Advance Data from Vital and Health Statistics* (280): 1–12. Hyattsville, Md.: National Center for Health Statistics, Division of Health Care Statistics.

Stone, Robyn, and others. 2002. *Promoting Quality in Nursing Homes: Evaluating the Wellspring Model—Final Report.* Report prepared for the Commonwealth Fund. Washington: American Association of Homes and Services for the Aging, Institute for the Future of Aging Studies.

Teno, Joan, and others. 1997. "The Early Impact of the Patient Self-Determination Act in Long-Term Care Facilities: Results from a Ten-State Sample." *Journal of the American Geriatrics Society* 45 (8): 939–44.

Tisdale, Sallie. 1988. "Harvest Moon: Portrait of a Nursing Home." *American Journal of Nursing* 88 (3): 296–300.

U.S. Department of Health and Human Services, Office of the Inspector-General. 1999a. *Abuse Complaints of Nursing Home Residents.* OEI-06-98-00340. Office of Evaluation and Inspections (May).

———. 1999b. *Quality of Care in Nursing Homes: An Overview.* Office of Evaluation and Inspections (March).

U.S. General Accounting Office. 1998. *California Nursing Homes: Care Problems Persist despite Federal and State Oversight.* GAO/HEHS-98-202. Report to the U.S. Senate Special Committee on Aging. Government Printing Office.

———. 1999a. *Nursing Homes: Additional Steps Needed to Strengthen Enforcement of Federal Quality Standards.* GAO/HEHS-99-46. Report to the U.S. Senate Special Committee on Aging. Government Printing Office.

———. 1999b. *Nursing Homes: Complaint Investigation Processes Often Inadequate to Protect Residents.* GAO/HEHS-99-80. Report to the U.S. Senate Special Committee on Aging. Government Printing Office.

———. 1999c. *Nursing Home Care: Enhanced HCFA Oversight of State Programs Would Better Ensure Quality.* GAO/HEHS-00-6. Report to the U.S. Senate Special Committee on Aging. Government Printing Office.

———. 2000. *Nursing Homes: Sustained Efforts Are Essential to Realize Potential of the Quality Initiatives.* GAO/HEHS-00-197. Report to the U.S. Senate Special Committee on Aging. Government Printing Office.

U.S. Senate Special Committee on Aging. 1998. *Betrayal: The Quality of Care in California Nursing Homes.* Committee Print 105-30 (July 21–28).

Wildfire, Judith, and others. 1997–98. "The Effect of Regulation on the Quality of Care in Board and Care Homes." *Generations* 21 (4): 25–29.

Williams, T. F., and Helena Temkin-Greener. 1996. "Older People, Dependency, and Trends in Supportive Care." In *The Future of Long-Term Care: Social and Policy Issues,* edited by R. H. Binstock, L. E. Cluff, and O. Von Mering, 51–74. Johns Hopkins University Press.

Zimmerman, David. 1998. "The Power of Information: Using Resident Assessment Data to Assure and Improve the Quality of Nursing Home Care." *Generations* 21 (4): 52–56.

12

Importance of Interdisciplinary Teams to Support Self-Care: The Example of Kaiser Permanente

Bruce Fireman

KAISER PERMANENTE HAS BEEN investing in disease management programs that provide evidence-based, patient-centered care for common chronic conditions. We are evaluating disease management programs for coronary artery disease, heart failure, diabetes, and persistent asthma during the years 1996 to 2001 in northern California, where Kaiser delivers health care to 3 million members, approximately 30 percent of the total population in this area. Eleven percent of Kaiser members are Medicare beneficiaries; 2 percent are Medicaid beneficiaries. The Kaiser population is diverse with respect to ethnicity: 13 percent Asian, 11 percent Latino, 8 percent African American, and 65 percent white. Founded in the 1940s, Kaiser Permanente has a long-standing commitment to health care that is comprehensive, integrated, prepaid, and not-for-profit.

Precursors of the disease management programs under evaluation were implemented at Kaiser in the early 1990s, part of the nationwide movement toward chronic care that is population based and evidence based and promotes patient self-care. Since 1998 Kaiser has more than doubled its investment in disease management programs in northern California to more than $45 million a year for seven programs that together fund about five hundred nursing-care managers and other staff. We are first evaluating the programs for which the most data are now available—the programs for coronary artery disease, heart failure, diabetes, and persistent asthma.

These programs share a common approach to disease management. Nonphysician care managers (usually nurses) manage medications and support patient self-care. The care managers are trained to use disease registries, linked clinical databases, protocols, and reminder systems to monitor patients, reach out to patients who are at high risk, and help ensure that care is consistent with evidence-based guidelines. The care managers are trained in how to motivate patients to maintain healthy life-styles and adhere to prescribed therapies. They make appropriate referrals to specialty care and community services. Patients communicate with the care managers in group visits and telephone visits more than in traditional one-on-one office visits.

These disease management programs promise a lot: they promise to improve the quality of care and reduce costs while making the care experience more satisfactory to patients and the practice of medicine more sustainable for physicians. The strategy has two key components: the use of technology and nonphysicians to "leverage" physicians and boost productivity and the use of risk stratification to target patients for whom the programs' services are expected to be cost-effective or cost-saving. The hope is that the costs of the disease management programs will be offset when morbidity among the targeted patients is averted.

Kaiser decided to invest in these programs for a number of reasons. First, in the public health and health services literature, there has been considerable support for this approach to chronic care.[1] Second, disease management programs draw upon and highlight Kaiser's historic strengths: proactive outreach to maintain health throughout the defined population for which Kaiser is accountable, integration of comprehensive health services across specialties and settings, use of information technology to improve care, and large-scale operations with infrastructure for financing and implementing innovative programs. Third, Kaiser's current marketplace strategy is to enhance its reputation as the "quality leader," expecting that consumers and purchasers will reward quality if it can be delivered at an affordable cost. Fourth, cost savings are promised without painful trade-offs that might compromise quality, or dissatisfy patients, or arouse resistance from physicians or other staff.

Is there evidence from Kaiser that these disease management programs are already delivering on their promise to improve the quality of chronic care and save costs? We have been examining variation—over time and across clinics—in measures of quality and cost in relation to variation in program implementation and enrollment. We assess whether trends are more favorable in areas that have had programs longer, committed more resources to the programs, and reached more of their target population. We are finding favorable trends in quality indicators, but we have not found cost savings.

Figure 12-1 shows recent trends in the prevalence of four chronic conditions at Kaiser in northern California from 1996 to 2000. The prevalence of diabetes has increased dramatically from 4.8 to 6.7 percent of Kaiser adults. Persistent

---

1. See Institute of Medicine Committee on Quality of Health Care in America (2001) and Wagner and others (2001).

Figure 12-1.   *Prevalence of Four Chronic Conditions, 1996–2000*

Incidence per 1,000 adults

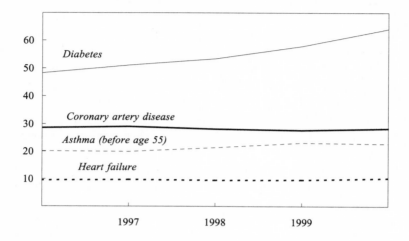

Source: Author's calculations based on data from the Kaiser Permanente Disease Management Program files.

asthma has increased from 2.0 to 2.3 percent, heart failure from 0.95 to 1.03 percent. The prevalence of coronary artery disease has decreased slightly. By the end of 2000 the programs for coronary artery disease, heart failure, diabetes, and asthma reached 35, 18, 18, and 13 percent, respectively, of all patients with the targeted conditions.

Figure 12-2 shows a sharp increase in the use of lipid-lowering medications among patients who have had a heart attack or a revascularization procedure; the corresponding improvement in lipid levels (LDLs) is illustrated in figure 12-3. Both graphs show favorable trends among the patients who enrolled in the disease management program and also in eligible patients who did not enroll. Enrollees fared better than nonenrollees in all the years from 1995 to 2001, but the gap between enrollees and nonenrollees steadily narrowed. The narrowing gap suggests that care management no longer improves lipid management as much as in the past, probably because more primary-care physicians now prescribe statins routinely and consistently to patients with coronary artery disease and hyperlipidemia. Perhaps some of the credit for this improvement in primary care can be attributed to the disease management programs and their champions. However, we did not find evidence of this when we examined variation across sixteen Kaiser medical centers in the timing and the extent of improvements in lipid control. The trends in lipid control are not

Figure 12-2.   *Use of Lipid-Lowering Drugs during Year after Heart Attack or Revascularization, Enrollees in the Disease Management Program and Eligible Nonenrollees, 1995–2001*

Percent using at least one drug

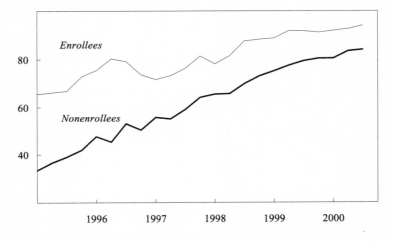

Source: Author's calculations based on data from the Kaiser Permanente Disease Management Program files.

strongly associated with the duration, scale, or reach of the disease management programs for coronary artery disease at the Kaiser medical centers.

Figure 12.4 shows improvement in asthma medication management. The use of anti-inflammatories increased dramatically while the use of beta-agonists declined. For asthma, we did find suggestive evidence that these trends were more favorable at the clinics that invested most in the program and where the programs reached the highest proportion of patients with persistent asthma.

Trends are also favorable in diabetics' glycemic and lipid control and in use of ACE inhibitors and beta-blockers among patients with heart failure, but the extent to which the improvement can be attributed to the disease management programs is not yet clear. From the available observational data in this "natural experiment" at Kaiser, it is reassuring to observe improvement in quality indicators but difficult to ascertain how much of the improvement would have occurred without the disease management programs.

For each of the four chronic conditions, we examined trends since 1996 in the utilization of health-care services and costs, comparing patients with each condition with health-plan members without the conditions who were similar

Figure 12-3.   *Mean Level of LDL during Year after Heart Attack or Revascularization, Enrollees in the Disease Management Program and Eligible Nonenrollees, 1995–2001*

Mean LDL value among those tested

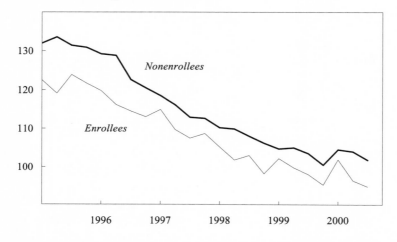

Source: Author's calculations based on data from the Kaiser Permanente Disease Management Program files.

in age and sex. Overall, trends in utilization and costs for patients with these chronic conditions were parallel to the trends for Kaiser members without these conditions. In general, with or without the chronic conditions, the results have included

—an increase in pharmacy utilization

—a slight increase in total clinic visits

—a shift in some clinic visits from physicians to other clinicians

—a decrease in emergency visits

—a slight increase in hospital stays and days

—an increase in overall costs

The trend has been more favorable for persistent asthma: emergency visits decreased substantially more in asthma patients than in similar patients without asthma, and hospital days for asthma decreased. Costs increased even for asthma, however. From 1996 to 2001, costs increased by 12.7, 11.4, 4.9, and 8.6 percent for patients with coronary artery disease, heart failure, diabetes, and asthma, respectively, after adjustment for the medical component of the consumer price index. It is possible that costs would have increased even more in the absence of disease management programs. However, we are also

Figure 12-4. *Annual Use of Anti-Inflammatories and Beta-Agonists by Patients with Persistent Asthma, 1995–2001*

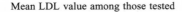
Mean LDL value among those tested

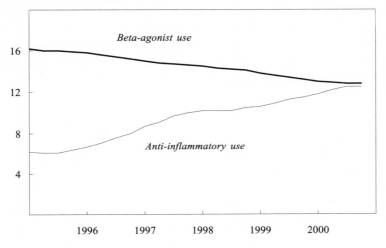

Source: Author's calculations based on data from the Kaiser Permanente Disease Management Program files.

examining several possible explanations for why these programs may not be saving costs, including the following:

—Program implementation was slower than anticipated. It takes more time and resources than anticipated to adapt information technology for tracking, targeting, and outreach.

—When physicians refer patients to these programs—and when patients self-refer—the programs' services are not targeted as well as anticipated; some program resources are diverted from the patients who need them most to those who want them most.

—Forecasts of the benefits of disease management over usual care did not anticipate improvements in usual care. To continuously improve on usual care, disease management programs must flexibly adjust to changes in the shortcomings of usual care.

—The hypothesized pathway—from disease management to guidelines-concordant care to reduced morbidity to cost savings—may be weaker or slower than anticipated. Expectations derived from reports written by disease management champions, based on data from "hothouse" pilot studies and clinical trials, may be unrealistic. Most health-care services that are cost-effective are not cost-saving.

Our evaluation of disease management programs at Kaiser Permanente is a work in progress; the findings to date are preliminary. Nevertheless, the early evidence from Kaiser suggests that disease management programs can contribute to rapid improvement in quality-of-care indicators, especially when effective well-tolerated medicines are available but have been underused; but that there may not be cost savings. Thus the promise of disease management programs should be articulated in terms of cost-effectiveness rather than cost savings.

References

Institute of Medicine Committee on Quality of Health Care in America. 2001. *Crossing the Quality Chasm.* Washington: National Academy Press.
Wagner, Edward H., and others. 2001. "Improving Chronic Illness Care: Translating Evidence into Action." *Health Affairs* 20 (6): 64–78.

13

Chronic-Care Initiatives: What We Have Learned and Implications for the Medicare Program

Marty Lynch, Carroll Estes, and Mauro Hernandez

G IVEN THE GROWING NUMBER of elderly and disabled Americans who receive health-care services through the Medicare program and the costs associated with their use of needed services, it is critical that we learn the best way to treat the chronic conditions faced by many of these beneficiaries. This paper reviews several sentinel initiatives that provide care to people with chronic conditions. It is not intended to be a comprehensive review of the literature; rather, we have selected a number of articles and initiatives that we believe contain important indicators of potential directions for Medicare in improving its approach to chronic care.

Types of chronic-care programs fall into three major categories. The first includes innovative federal and state programs, which attempt to integrate medical, home, and community-based services for the people with chronic conditions. Some of the best-known programs of this type are the Program of All-Inclusive Care for the Elderly (PACE), the first- and second-generation social health maintenance organizations (SHMOs), and state-sponsored initiatives for Medicare and Medicaid eligibles, such as Minnesota Senior Health Options (MSHO).

A second major category includes disease management programs, which attempt to improve medical management of chronic disease. Examples of these programs include the Breakthrough Series Best Practice Collaborative approach to chronic-disease care being conducted in a number of health-care systems, including community health centers.[1] Another example related to chronic medical management is the group-clinic approach for patients suffering from chronic diseases practiced in some regions by Kaiser Permanente.[2]

---

1. Ellrodt and others (1997); Katon and others (1995); McCulloch and others (1998); Wagner, Glasgow, and others (2001).
2. Sadur and others (1999).

Yet another is the emphasis on teaching self-care included in many of the disease management programs.[3]

A third category is the high-risk care-management approach developed by a number of managed-care organizations and medical groups to identify high-risk members and provide special care management in an effort to improve care in general and control high utilization and expenditures.[4] Improvements in functional status and reductions in hospitalization costs have also been reported by nursing homes and managed-care organizations that employ geriatric nurse practitioners (GNPs) to work collaboratively with primary-care physicians of these more impaired long-term-care residents.[5]

All of these approaches rely on some ability to track information about patients, their diagnoses, and utilization. Ideally, such information can allow physicians and other providers to better follow patients with chronic conditions and link actual care delivery to evidence-based protocols.[6]

Methodology

Articles were selected based on keyword, title, and author searches, using academic databases, including PubMed and MedLine, of chronic-care management programs, with preference given to peer-reviewed articles reporting quantifiable results. Additional reports were found using Internet search engines and searches on selected websites such as the AARP Research Center, the National Academy for State Health Policy, the University of Maryland Medicare-Medicaid Integration Program, the Urban Institute, and others. A snowball approach was then used to locate additional references identified in articles from the initial search. Interviews with several key informants were completed to provide their perspectives on innovations in chronic-care programs, barriers faced by those programs, and implications for the Medicare programs. Because extensive interviewing was beyond the scope of this project, several key informants were chosen based upon recommendations from National Academy of Social Insurance staff and our own identification of researchers with recognized expertise in chronic-disease management, care management and coordination, integrated medical and long-term-care initiatives, and health maintenance organization practices and performance. The

3. Lorig and others (1999); Norris, Engelgau, and Narayan (2001).
4. Boult and others (2001); Boult, Pualwan, and others (1998); Quinn, Prybylo, and Pannone (1999).
5. Buchanan and others (1990); Burl and others (1998).
6. Baker and others (2001); Schraeder, Britt, and Shelton (2000).

combination of literature review and key informant interviews was used to perform a basic meta-analysis of the field.

Federal Demonstrations

The Program of All-Inclusive Care for the Elderly (PACE) has approximately twenty years of experience fully integrating medical, home-based, and community-based care in a small managed-care model for elders with severe chronic conditions.[7] All participants must meet nursing-home admission requirements in their state and thus have significant functional activity of daily living (ADL) problems as well as several chronic-disease problems. Program participants receive intensive care coordination provided by a multidisciplinary team, which includes the PACE primary-care physician, social worker, physical, speech, and occupational therapists as well as nursing, activity, and transportation staff.[8] Most PACE members attend an adult day health center located within a primary-care clinic and receive the majority of their medical and community-based services in that setting. Services are also provided in participants' homes. The programs typically contract with outside entities for hospital and medical specialty services but retain control both through reimbursement methods and through primary-care physician management of utilization.

Payment incentives in the program support coordination of care and substitution of primary and basic home and community care for high-cost acute care. The programs are required to provide basic Medicare and Medicaid services but may also choose to use other less typical interventions.[9] One takes its members on fishing trips and has a small drama group, which performs at local events.[10] The programs often are able to avoid or shorten hospital stays by substituting intensive services from the rest of the team for hospital care.[11] Programs also have great flexibility in funding educational or preventive activities. They are able to make decisions based on the individual patient's care plan and overall budget constraints. Given the wide range of medical and long-term risk accepted by the programs, they manage greater numbers of dollars than most managed-care programs and have additional flexibility to

---

7. Eng and others (1997).

8. Shannon and Van Reenen (1998); Zimmerman, Pemberton, and Thomas (1998).

9. Eng and others (1997).

10. Peter Szutu, CEO of Center for Elders' Independence, personal communication with authors, Oakland, Calif.

11. Eng and others (1997).

fund preventive or community-based interventions.[12] The programs make efforts to involve members and their families in the care-planning and coordination process. Some continue to use family members as enrollees' caregivers. Both physical and cognitive disabilities are significant in PACE programs and may make participant empowerment and control a challenge.[13]

Slow growth—there are perhaps only ten thousand members nationwide—has limited the impact and significance of the program.[14] Nonetheless, PACE is a Medicare benefit recognized in the Balanced Budget Act of 1997 and continues to grow.[15] It is also subject to state-to-state variations based on individual states' willingness to process PACE applications or negotiate the Medicaid portion of the capitation payment, given concerns about the high cost of providing the benefit. Despite these issues, PACE continues to be one of the few successful models for integrating the full range of medical and chronic-care services across both the Medicare and Medicaid programs. Reported positive outcomes include, "steady census growth, good consumer satisfaction, reduction in use of institutional care, controlled utilization of medical services, and cost savings to public and private payers of care, including Medicare and Medicaid."[16]

The Social Health Maintenance Organization (SHMO) has provided a federally supported model for adding a limited chronic-care benefit, which can cover a range of home- and community-based-care services, to a Medicare health maintenance organization (HMO) structure. Four first-generation SHMOs experienced mixed success in the 1980s. For the most part, the SHMO I sites were able to manage utilization of home- and community-based care by using care coordinators to design a care plan and authorize services for disabled members but experienced greater difficulty reaching enrollment targets and managing hospital utilization.[17] Utilization was especially problematic for those early SHMO sites that were not based in an existing HMO and did not have existing practices in place to control high-cost utilization.[18] They also were criticized for favorable enrollment and disenrollment practices and lack of day-to-day coordination between physicians and care coordinators.[19]

12. Eng and others (1997).
13. Branch, Coulam, and Zimmerman (1995).
14. Branch and others (1995); Kane, Illston, and Miller (1992).
15. Irvin, Massey, and Dorsey (1997).
16. Eng and others (1997, p. 223).
17. Newcomer and others (1995).
18. Harrington and Newcomer (1991).
19. Harrington, Newcomer, and Preston (1993); Harrington, Lynch, and Newcomer (1993).

Second-generation SHMOs attempted to apply risk-adjustment payment methodology to discourage favorable selection as well as further geriatric innovation and integration of care.[20] Only one health plan (Health Plan of Nevada) was added in the second generation of the SHMO program, owing to disagreement on the risk-adjusted payment methodology.[21] The SHMOs use care coordinators to work with high-risk or disabled members. High-risk members are identified either through a screening instrument or by physician referral. Available services include standard Medicare benefits plus home- and community-care-based services within the limits of the SHMO benefit structure. These services could include personal assistance, transportation, durable medical equipment, home modification, or other services. Members who need long-term nursing-home care were disenrolled from the SHMO I demonstration. The SHMO II plan continues enrollment for members who need nursing-home care but are not at risk for skilled-nursing-facility costs. In the SHMO I, approximately 5 percent of members were targeted for special chronic-care services while in the lone operative SHMO II site approximately 20 percent receive some level of care coordination or monitoring.[22] The second-generation SHMOs have also encouraged formal involvement of geriatricians in the care-planning process.[23]

The second-generation SHMOs are subject to basic managed-care incentives similar to any Medicare HMO. They must control high-cost utilization but may be able to authorize additional basic services that substitute for more costly care. Utilization and management procedures are also consistent with Medicare HMO practice. The most recent report to the Health Care Financing Administration (HCFA)[24] on the SHMO demonstration suggests that significant outcomes (as compared with Medicare Plus Choice HMOs) related to utilization, health status, and slowing decline in functional ability have not been identified. In addition, the report suggests that two of the remaining three SHMO I sites are receiving more additional revenues from the Centers for Medicare and Medicaid Services (CMS) because of their special payment methodology than they are spending on care coordination and home- and community-based services. The report recommends that the SHMO demonstration be phased out or transitioned either to a standard Medicare Plus Choice format or to a risk-adjusted payment method used in the one SHMO II plan.

20. Kane and others (1997).
21. Newcomer, Harrington, and Kane (2000).
22. Newcomer (2001).
23. Kane and others (1997).
24. Wooldridge and others (2001).

State Efforts Targeting Dual Eligibles

Several states have established initiatives that attempt to integrate medical and chronic long-term care for their Medicare- and Medicaid-eligible population in single health plans.[25] Financial and operational integration for these programs is difficult without a Medicare waiver, given beneficiaries' ability to freely choose to either enroll in a managed-care plan or remain in a traditional fee-for-service Medicare plan.[26] The State of Minnesota has established Minnesota Senior Health Options (MSHO), which enables Medicaid funds to be blended with Medicare dollars through a Medicare waiver allowing health plans to integrate delivery and financing of a full range of medical and chronic long-term-care services in a number of health plans made available to beneficiaries.[27] The MSHO program includes case management services for high-risk patients as well as financial incentives to encourage the use of home- and community-based services and early nursing-home discharges.[28]

A number of other states (Massachusetts, Florida, Texas, Wisconsin, Oregon, for example) have tried to establish initiatives for the elderly using a variety of mechanisms such as Medicaid Home and Community Based Waiver programs.[29] Texas Star Plus uses concurrent Medicaid 1915(b) and 1915(c) waivers to provide acute- and long-term-care services to disabled and elderly Medicaid beneficiaries, with Medicare enrollment in one of the plans being voluntary with an enriched benefit structure serving as an incentive. These programs typically rely on care coordination services to achieve integration between acute- and long-term-care services.[30]

Any of these approaches may also provide preventive health education aimed at the management of chronic disease. Providers may also use chronic-disease management protocols, but the main intervention is the effort to integrate acute medical and chronic long-term-care services through the combined use of Medicare for acute services and Medicaid for home- and community-based-care services, often with a case manager helping facilitate the care.[31] Whether the participating health plans or physicians use clinical-disease

25. Coleman and others (1999); National Chronic Care Consortium (2001).

26. Wiener and Stevenson (1998).

27. National Chronic Care Consortium (2001).

28. Kane, Kane, and Ladd (1998); Robyn Stone, "Long-Term Care for the Elderly with Disabilities: Current Policy, Emerging Trends, and Implications for the Twenty-First Century" (www.milbank.org/0008stone/ [December 5, 2000]).

29. Coleman (1998); Mollica and Riley (1997).

30. Wiener and Stevenson (1998).

31. Mollica and Riley (1997).

management protocols is probably variable. Similarly, the level of utilization and management procedures will depend on whether the participating plan or provider is at risk for the whole range of services, such as in the PACE demonstration, or only for Medicaid services when dual-eligible beneficiaries do not choose to enroll in the same Medicare plan, thus splitting the financing for medical and long-term-care services. Although these state demonstrations attempt to align incentives between the Medicare and Medicaid programs, for the most part there remain perverse incentives for states to maximize expenditures borne by the Medicare program and for Medicare providers to shift costs to Medicaid.[32] For example, nursing homes paid for by Medicaid may have little incentive to manage acute episodes of chronic conditions without simply sending the resident to the hospital, which will be covered by Medicare. States may also require nursing homes to become certified under Medicare as well as Medicaid in order to shift some costs to Medicare.[33]

Chronic-Care Coordination Programs

Mathematica contracted with HCFA in an effort to study successful programs for the coordination of care in chronic illness and recommend design options for fee-for-service Medicare beneficiaries.[34] They identified these programs as "serving chronically ill persons 'at risk' for adverse outcomes and expensive care" by "(1) identifying those medical, functional, social, and emotional needs that increase their risk of adverse health events; (2) addressing those needs through education in self-care, optimization of medical treatment, and integration of care fragmented by setting or provider; and (3) monitoring patients for progress and early signs of problems."[35] They further delineated case management programs, which target high-risk patients with costly utilization and complex medical and social problems, and disease management programs, which focus on a specific major chronic problem such as diabetes or congestive heart failure, even though the recipient of services may have additional chronic problems. Disease management programs tended to have more specific guidelines and procedures and use information technology to help with feedback and management. Emphasis was on building relationships with patients, education of patients, and monitoring care for compliance with

32. Wiener and Stevenson (1998).
33. Mollica and Riley (1997); Wiener and Stevenson (1998).
34. Chen and others (2000).
35. Chen and others (2000, p. xiii).

protocols. Case management programs were more likely to cover medical, functional, social, and emotional issues.[36]

Financial incentives for both types of programs would seem to favor their implementation in organizations that bear some risk for high-cost patients, including health plans, medical groups that share risk with health plans, and hospitals that either share risk or bear risk for length and cost of hospital stays under the diagnosis-related group reimbursement system. One randomized controlled trial measuring the effects of a social-work-oriented case management model found no significant reduction in health care costs for older Medicare Plus Choice enrollees.[37] Similar findings were reported for three other HCFA-funded case management demonstrations for high-cost fee-for-service Medicare beneficiaries with no improvements in self-care, health, or Medicare spending.[38] However, the authors of this study recommend investigating other models with more physician involvement, goal-orientation, and financial incentives tied to cost savings.

Physician-led and nurse-managed models of case management seem to report better outcomes, particularly those that are disease oriented. For postmyocardial infarction patients, such case management efforts have been found to be "considerably more effective than usual medical care for modification of coronary risk factors after myocardial infarction" and able to significantly reduce psychological-distress risk factors, such as anxiety and anger.[39] Similarly, programs involving case management by nurses in group-model HMOs have reported improved management and control of diabetes.[40] Case management services provided through the Medicare Alzheimer's disease demonstration were shown to be protective against nursing-home placement and hospitalization, to have a tendency toward reduced health-care expenditures, and to significantly reduce unmet needs without reducing informal caregiving.[41]

One asthma disease management program was shown to reduce emergency visit rates and result in projected Medicaid savings of "$3 to $4 for every incremental dollar spent providing disease management support to physicians."[42] A 1999 review of sixteen studies conducted from 1983 to 1998 reports that heart failure disease management programs "appear to be a cost-effective

36. Chen and others (2000, p. xvii–xix).
37. Boult and others (2000).
38. Schore, Brown, and Cheh (1999).
39. DeBusk and others (1994, p. 721); Taylor and others (1997).
40. Aubert and others (1998); Sikka and others (1999).
41. Newcomer, Arnsberger, and Zhang (1997); Newcomer and others (1999); Yordi and others (1997).
42. Rossiter and others (2000, 188).

approach to reducing morbidity and enhancing quality of life in selected patients with heart failure."[43] However, the effectiveness and reach of the more innovative chronic-disease management programs is reportedly limited "by their reliance on traditional patient education, rather than modern self-management support, poor linkages to primary care, and reliance on referrals rather than population-based approaches."[44]

Other Noteworthy Chronic-Disease Management Initiatives

The Kaiser Permanente system has initiated a number of chronic-disease management programs in regions around the country. Kaiser Northern California has instituted tiered chronic-disease programs for several different chronic conditions.[45] These interventions include interdisciplinary teams and self-care teaching through motivational interviewing and use evidence-based clinical guidelines, disease registries, clinical databases, and assessment tools to help assess and manage behavioral and social problems. Kaiser also uses population-based approaches to reminder systems and outreach to patients overdue for exams and visits. Group visits and telephone monitoring are also used. These interventions are not limited to Medicare Plus Choice plan members.

Kaiser also identifies a continuum of care management activities for its heart failure patients, including intensive management for the most complex patients, care management for those with moderate risk, and self-management based on education classes and outreach for lower-risk patients. Initial findings on clinical management indicators and patient satisfaction have improved during the project.[46] The program also is aimed at reducing overall utilization and inappropriate utilization as well as shifting more work to less costly care providers, including teams using improved technology to increase their productivity.

The Group Health Cooperative of Puget Sound, a staff-model HMO, tested a population-based chronic-care model that combined a number of chronic-disease interventions, including an online registry of diabetic patients, evidence-based guidelines for clinical screening and management, support for patient self-management, group visits for diabetics, and diabetic expertise available to primary-care teams.[47] Results indicated improved clinical testing outcomes, as well as improved patient and provider satisfaction.

43. Rich (1999).
44. Wagner and others (1999).
45. Fireman, Carpenter, and Bartlett (2000).
46. Fireman, Carpenter, and Bartlett (2000).
47. McCulloch and others (1998).

A number of health systems have instituted group or cluster visits, during which a number of patients are seen together in a single session, for patients with diabetes or other chronic diseases.[48] Group visits have been used with both Medicare- and non-Medicare-covered users. Edward Wagner and colleagues studied the impact of these chronic-care group visits on process and outcome of diabetic care in a staff-model HMO. The intervention included half-day chronic-care clinics for approximately eight patients. The group visits included standard assessments, visits with the primary-care physician, nurse, and a clinical pharmacist as well as a group-education and peer-support meeting. The study indicated a positive association with patient satisfaction and a number of clinical outcomes supporting the potential positive role of the group-visit approach with chronic-disease patients.[49] Arne Beck and colleagues found that monthly group visits for older patients with high utilization and at least one chronic condition reduced emergency-room use, repeat hospital admissions, physician visits, and overall costs ($14.79 a month, on average, for each participant) while increasing nurse visits, calls, and patient and physician satisfaction.[50] These findings were consistent with a later study of older patients showing reduced emergency-room use.[51] Another study targeting older clients at risk of hospitalization or experiencing functional decline also found high levels of patient satisfaction; however, significantly improved outcomes for selected geriatric syndromes (urinary incontinence, falls, depression, impairment of physical functioning, the need for high-risk medication prescriptions) were not demonstrated.[52]

The Breakthrough Series Best Practice Collaborative approach, combined with the Chronic Care Model developed by the Group Health Cooperative in Puget Sound, was used to improve care for chronic illness in a variety of organizations, including academic medical centers, hospital-based programs, health plans, community health centers, and other safety-net providers.[53] Early efforts were aimed at diabetes management; additional collaboratives worked on improving care for congestive heart failure, depression, and asthma as well.

These collaborative efforts emphasized learning sessions focused on evidence-based interventions followed by implementation in pilot sites and follow-up activities such as e-mail, personal visits, phone assessment, and website use. Interventions focused on clinical information systems such as

48. Beck and others (1997); Sadur and others (1999).
49. Wagner, Grothaus, and others (2001).
50. Beck and others (1997).
51. Coleman and others (2001).
52. Coleman and others (1999).
53. Wagner, Glasgow, and others (2001).

registry data, decision support mechanisms such as flow sheets with guidelines and referral guidelines, change in delivery of services such as the use of nurse managers and group visits, support for case management, links to community resources, and development of organizational supports for pilot sites. Most of the participating sites experienced improvements in clinical processes and in care outcomes, with community health centers experiencing some of the largest improvements. One other collaborative primary-care-practice model for community-based elderly persons in Illinois reported significantly reduced mortality rates for the treatment group in the second year of the study without increased hospital utilization.[54]

A number of the initiatives discussed involve patient self-care management interventions. It is possible to provide a general prevention or wellness-oriented program outside of normal medical or health plan settings. Suzanne Leveille and colleagues describe a Health Enhancement Program (HEP) model building off earlier preventive efforts based in a senior center.[55] The older participants in the HEP model attained positive outcomes in reduced hospital utilization and less decline in function when compared with a control group by using nurse and social-worker education on health issues, including chronic care, health goal setting for participants, and exercise program participation. Net annual savings of approximately $1,200 for each participant were identified. The intervention cost approximately $300.[56] This intervention is currently being replicated in senior-housing facilities, in a homeless-senior program, and with long-term-care insurance purchasers of the CalPERS program.[57]

Targeting Residents in Long-Term-Care Settings

We found a limited number of chronic-care studies targeting Medicare beneficiaries living in long-term-care settings such as nursing homes, assisted-living facilities, or residential care. There has been some interest in the role of GNPs employed by nursing homes, with early studies showing reduced hospital service admissions and use, some favorable changes in ADL measures, a substitution effect for physician care, reductions in hospital admission rates and total hospital days, and no significant adverse effect on nursing-home costs or profits.[58] One interview-based study finds only differences in hospital

54. Quinn and others (1999).
55. Leveille and others (1998); Health Enhancement Program (HEP).
56. Leveille and others (1998).
57. California HealthCare Foundation (2001).
58. Kane and others (1989); Buchanan and others (1990); Burl and Bonner (1991); Joseph and Boult (1998).

admission rates between newly admitted nursing-home residents with a GNP and those without a GNP.[59] Shorter hospital stays have also been shown for hospitalized nursing-home patients when comanaged by a GNP-physician team within the acute-care setting.[60]

Few of the largest Medicare risk-contracting HMOs with the largest Medicare-beneficiary enrollment levels have formal primary-care programs for nursing-home residents.[61] A related Medicare HMO alternative to this approach is the EverCare model, which serves nursing-home residents who are either Medicare-only beneficiaries or dually eligible nursing-home residents.[62] EverCare operates through Medicare and Medicaid waivers and is currently participating in an HCFA demonstration project in six states, as well as through other local health plans in three other states.[63] EverCare is based on a collaborative team approach involving a primary-care physician and a GNP, an approach that provides more intensive on-site primary care to frail elderly nursing-home patients under a capitated Medicare-covered package of services.[64] Although the HCFA evaluations have not been completed, savings from shorter hospital stays have been realized by purchasing more services from the participating nursing homes and by minimizing hospitalization.[65] Further development of this model among HMOs may be limited by problems recruiting GNPs and physicians as well as limited research results (see table 13-1).[66]

Beneficiary Empowerment Issues in Chronic Care

Beneficiary empowerment has been brought squarely into health policy in four ways: disability advocates promoting the independent-living movement and the Americans with Disabilities Act (ADA), for which consumer direction and empowerment are cornerstone principles;[67] research evidence on the import of behavioral and environmental risk factors and work of the assistant secretary for health and the surgeon general in setting national health promo-

59. Garrard and others (1990).
60. Miller (1997).
61. Farley and others (1999).
62. Kane and others (1998).
63. Stone, "Long-Term Care for the Elderly with Disabilities"; EverCare, "Health Care Programs" (www.myevercare.com/About_Us/about_us.html [October 6, 2001]).
64. Ryan (1999); Kane and Huck (2000).
65. Kane and others (1998); Malone, Chase, and Bayard (1993).
66. Fama and Fox (1997).
67. Wiener and others (2001).

Table 13-1. *Current Chronic-Care Initiative Models*

Characteristic	Medical long-term-care integration programs	Care management programs	Disease management programs	Residential programs
Target population	SNF eligible Dual eligible Frail elders	High-cost users	Major chronic disease	Major chronic disease
Interventions	Medical and long-term care Care coordination Multidisciplinary team	Risk assessment Needs assessment Care planning Service arrangement Monitoring	Registry Self-care education and support Group visits Evidence-based protocols	Primary-care physician and geriatric nurse practitioner team Intensive primary-care management
Medicare benefits	Acute medical only	In some Medicare + Choice programs	Some interventions can be covered	Acute medical covered
Financing model	Medicare, Medicaid Medicare premiums Risk-based capitation	HMO, medical group Special program	Health plan, medical group, medical center, hospital	Medicare or Medicaid demonstration
Strengths	Controlled expenditures compared with skilled-nursing facility Reduced hospital days	Some cost and utilization control	Improved clinical measures Increased patient satisfaction	Initial reduction of hospital days
Weaknesses	Small numbers enrolled Waiver process difficult Medicare enrollment Voluntary	Cost-control oriented versus functionally oriented Limited applicability to small fee-for-service providers	Small numbers to date Requires organizational supports and information systems May be difficult to implement in small practices or nongroup HMOs	Demonstration Most skilled-nursing facilities not at risk for hospital Requires waiver

tion and disease prevention goals;[68] research on inequality and health high-lighting the independent effects on health of social factors such as race and racism;[69] and work on the "medicalization" of social problems[70] that points to many potentially modifiable nonmedical factors that are key to these problems. Estes and Binney discuss the biomedicalization of aging, whereby normal aging processes are constructed in medical terms with control of these pro-cesses shifting to the medical profession or health-care industry and rendering the patient more dependent and powerless.[71] Increasing privatization and rationalization of health-care delivery also shifts the domain of caring for the elderly into the business sector, where financial and bureaucratic (for example, managed-care) interests play a dominant role, with potentially disempowering effects on consumers.[72]

Arguments for the "empowerment imperative" for the disabled, chronically ill, and elderly have been made not only on political and ideological grounds but also with the knowledge that the acute-care model is woefully inadequate (and too expensive) to the task of dealing with the largely social-supportive and personal-care needs of millions of these individuals.[73] Given the sociodemographics of aging and chronic disease, the nation can ill afford to "produce" more (or new) dependencies in patients because of what we do and do not finance and what is excluded from coverage (for example, reimbursement limits on reha-bilitation and prevention). Under the paradigm of patient passivity and compli-ance, there is a risk that health policy may actually contribute to the unneces-sary dependency of the chronically ill by what it does not cover. This could be a form of iatrogenically produced dependency.

Many of the chronic-care initiatives described earlier, whether integrating acute-care and long-term chronic-care services or improving disease manage-ment for a specific condition, are placed in capitated health-plan settings or in academic or hospital settings subject to financial utilization incentives. From a beneficiary point of view, these incentives raise questions as to whether the interests of the beneficiary take precedence over the financial interests of the health plan, hospital, or medical center.[74] Ideally, the chronic-disease initia-tives discussed above could combine the best interests of both: the use of flexible financing to support preventive and self-care activities while saving

68. U.S. Department of Health and Human Services (1998).
69. Collins and Williams (1999).
70. Conrad and Schneider (1992).
71. Estes and Binney (1989).
72. Estes and others (2001).
73. Estes, Casper, and Binney (1993).
74. Bodenheimer (2000).

dollars spent on inappropriate utilization. Despite earlier beliefs that consumer control was primarily an issue for younger disabled people, recent survey data suggest that even among elderly consumers, a significant and growing number would prefer some level of control over the services they receive.[75] We did not find data on the relative involvement of for-profit and nonprofit health plans or health systems in these innovative programs. The initiatives described do, however, indicate the involvement of the large nonprofit health plans such as Kaiser and Group Health. Consumers might rightly fear bottom-line motivation facing for-profit systems unless regulatory controls assured appropriate chronic-care management in all Medicare-funded settings.

Implications for Medicare

There is at least some evidence, noted earlier, that all of the initiatives described above have had some success, whether it be the ability of the specialized plans like PACE, SHMOs, and the dual-eligible programs to stay in business while managing a complex set of patient needs, the improvement of clinical outcomes and processes as measured in chronic-disease collaboratives, or improvements in patient and provider satisfaction. Given successes to date, we can ask how these models could be extended to additional Medicare beneficiaries. Certainly many of the disease management interventions can be delivered under existing regulations by Medicare Plus Choice programs. It is much more difficult for fee-for-service Medicare providers to deliver care management, group visits, self-care management training, and other potentially helpful services under existing regulations.

Existing chronic-care initiatives focus on linking acute medical care to home- and community-based services or on expanding medical services to include education, self-care management, case management, and population-based clinical improvements. Approaches aimed at chronic long-term-care services, care management with high-cost users, and specific disease management programs do not necessarily intersect. There is little evidence of cross-initiative planning in place to date, and it is probably safe to assume that few Medicare beneficiaries receive state-of-the-art care across a range of functional and disease management needs.

Another challenging question is posed by the paucity of initiatives that reach private providers or small physician groups providing care under the traditional fee-for-service Medicare program. Chronic-condition collaborative participants and demonstration participants, with a few exceptions, have been

75. Coleman (2001).

medical centers, health plans, hospitals, safety-net providers, community health centers, and others with some level of infrastructure, not small private providers. This is also true for most programs that integrate medical, home-, and community-based services. Most initiative approaches of both types require organizational support and resources, including somewhat sophisticated information systems.[76] Group- and staff-model plans, which have birthed a number of the initiatives discussed above, are more likely to be able to influence their physicians, as well as provide necessary structural supports, than plans that shift risk to independent practice association structures. Incentives related to the ability to experience cost savings from reduced utilization of hospital days may also be important in systems implementing these initiatives and are present in health plans, hospitals, and medical centers.

Given that the majority of initiatives discussed here have taken place in managed-care settings, and that organizational structure, information systems, and financial incentives are better aligned to support disease management in health plans, can we not presume that supporting the growth of managed care in Medicare might also create a favorable climate for chronic-disease management? On the other hand, the Medicare Plus Choice program is extremely volatile at this point in time: plans have pulled out of the business or out of specific geographic areas. In 2001, 934,000 (13.6 percent of Medicare Plus Choice members) were displaced from their plans.[77] It is unclear whether Congress will concede to the plans' complaints and raise payment rates significantly, perhaps leading to enrollment growth, or whether enrollment will continue to plummet as plans are withdrawn from the market. Medicare Plus Choice programs have also not yet shown an interest in adding functionally oriented chronic- and long-term-care services to their products. Medicare Plus Choice probably does provide a favorable environment for disease management programs, given the presence of necessary infrastructure and incentives to control overall costs. Plan behavior and geographic location may also be critical factors in the availability of disease management programs, suggesting that regulatory requirements and uniform program expectations throughout Medicare may be critical in assuring that beneficiaries have equitable access to proven chronic-care initiatives.

Recommendations

These factors may make it difficult to plan for translating successes of existing initiatives into traditional Medicare used by millions of older and

76. Luft (2001).
77. Stuber, Dallek, and Biles (2001).

disabled Americans. Nonetheless, Medicare has begun to make the transition to paying for additional preventive and educational services (immunizations, mammograms, and diabetes education, to name a few). Below are a number of recommendations for improvements to the Medicare program, which would allow improved chronic-care management.

Short-Term Methods to Bring Initiative Benefits to the Medicare Fee-for-Service Population

A number of care management programs have used risk assessment to identify members in order to target special chronic-care services.[78] The Centers for Medicare and Medicaid Services should identify high-risk Medicare beneficiaries or provide incentives for primary-care physicians to do so, using standard screening instruments now used by health plans or through participating physician referral. Once high-risk patients have been identified, beneficiaries with serious chronic diseases can be made eligible for case management services paid for by Medicare.

Information system infrastructure may present a problem for non–health plan providers. Health plans, medical centers, hospitals, and community health centers that have participated in chronic-disease collaboratives all have some capability to use their information systems to build disease registries. The CMS could provide basic software to private providers and small medical groups— in essence, allowing them to easily build chronic-disease registries for their practices in programs like Access or Excel.[79]

Given the scarcity of chronic-disease initiatives in fee-for-service Medicare, independent primary-care providers or small groups of providers could be offered reimbursement to participate in collaborative training models focusing on chronic-disease care. These could be centered regionally or could use teleconferencing capabilities or Internet-based distance-learning tools present in many communities to avoid cost and time of travel. Given positive outcomes associated with a number of chronic-disease interventions,[80] Medicare program expectations should be fostered for all providers to use evidence-based chronic-disease interventions and use Medicare professional review organizations to help publicize these guidelines, monitor providers, and build support systems for providers in implementing guidelines.

---

78. Quinn and others (1999); Rich and others (1995); Boult, Boult, and others (1998); Boult and others (2001).

79. Wagner (2001); Luft (2001).

80. Knox and Mischke (1999); Rich (1999); Rossiter and others (2000); Rubin, Dietrich, and Hawk (1998).

The Medicare fee-for-service payment methodology should be made flexible enough to encourage group-visit models for chronic-disease care and encourage providers to use these visits as part of their chronic-disease program. These measures should include reimbursement for nursing and for nutritionist services provided in these programs.

Making It Easier for States to Improve Chronic Care and Integrate with Medicare

A major problem in integrating acute and chronic care is the split between Medicare and Medicaid coverage and incentives for state and federal governments to shift costs from one payer to the other.[81] Yet obtaining waivers to link these two reimbursement streams has been extremely difficult and has often taken many years. Therefore, we recommend that states be encouraged by CMS to offer voluntary enrollment in health plans that link Medicaid and Medicare dollars for acute-care integrated with home- and community-based services for dual eligibles with chronic conditions—without requiring waivers or placing difficult regulatory barriers on cooperating plans, such as separate health-plan certification processes for both Medicare and Medicaid.

Medicare Plus Choice

Some Medicare Plus Choice programs have implemented disease management programs with a number of positive outcomes, as noted above. We suggest that the CMS make evidence-based chronic-disease management a program expectation for Medicare Plus Choice contractors and consider payment incentives for those plans that show improved chronic-disease process and outcome measures.

Educating Medicare Beneficiaries

Growing numbers of consumers have indicated a preference for some control over the services they receive. Self-care education has also been an important part of disease management approaches. We would recommend that the CMS initiate a beneficiary-education program, using major elder and disabled advocacy organizations, insurance counseling programs, and foundation-sponsored programs like the Center for Medicare Education to develop user-friendly materials about chronic-disease self-care, necessary clinical

81. Wiener and Stevenson (1998).

testing, and advice for interacting with their physician or health plan. Beneficiaries should also be educated about consumer rights and the Medicare appeals processes.

Long Term: Medicare Plus Choice

Health plans have expressed concerns that special chronic-care programs might encourage sicker beneficiaries to enroll. The CMS should continue to develop risk adjustment models which would, in essence, pay health plans to enroll members with chronic-disease problems while avoiding problems of adverse selection.[82]

Continuing Research

Because there is no consensus on the specifics of chronic-disease management protocols, the CMS should fund additional real-time research on a variety of care management, wellness, disease management, and chronic-care integration programs in large-scale naturally occurring settings not requiring randomized designs. Such research should also identify racial and socioeconomic disparities in the use of these initiatives and the outcomes produced by them. Randomized trials present difficulties for health plans and provider groups.[83]

Integrate Chronic and Acute Care in Medicare

In the long run, the CMS should work toward integrating home- and community-based-care services responding to the functional needs of beneficiaries with chronic conditions into the Medicare program to avoid cost shifting between the Medicare and Medicaid programs and to improve quality and accessibility of care for consumers with chronic problems.

References

Aubert, R. E., and others. 1998. "Nurse Case Management to Improve Glycemic Control in Diabetic Patients in a Health Maintenance Organization: A Randomized, Controlled Trial." *Annals of Internal Medicine* 129 (8): 605–12.

Baker, A. M., and others. 2001. "A Web-Based Diabetes Care Management Support System." *Joint Commission Journal on Quality Improvement* 27 (4): 179–90.

82. Newcomer (2001); Luft (2001).
83. Fox (2001).

Beck, A., and others. 1997. "A Randomized Trial of Group Outpatient Visits for Chronically Ill Older HMO Members: The Cooperative Health Care Clinic." *Journal of the American Geriatric Society* 45 (5): 543–49.

Bodenheimer, T. 2000. "Disease Management in the American Market." *British Medical Journal* 320 (7234): 563–66.

Boult, C., L. Boult, and others. 1998. "Outpatient Geriatric Evaluation and Management." *Journal of the American Geriatric Society* 46 (3): 296–302.

Boult, C., T. F. Pualwan, and others. 1998. "Identification and Assessment of High-Risk Seniors: HMO Workgroup on Care Management." *American Journal of Managed Care* 4 (8): 1137–46.

Boult, C., and others. 2000. "The Effect of Case Management on the Costs of Health Care for Enrollees in Medicare Plus Choice Plans: A Randomized Trial." *Journal of the American Geriatric Society* 48 (8): 996–1001.

Boult, C., and others. 2001. "A Randomized Clinical Trial of Outpatient Geriatric Evaluation and Management." *Journal of the American Geriatric Society* 49 (4): 351–59.

Branch, L. G., R. F. Coulam, and Y. A. Zimmerman. 1995. "The PACE Evaluation: Initial Findings." *Gerontologist* 35 (3): 349–59.

Buchanan, J. L., and others. 1990. "Assessing Cost Effects of Nursing-Home-Based Geriatric Nurse Practitioners." *Health Care Finance Review* 11 (3): 67–78.

Burl, J. B., and A. F. Bonner. 1991. "A Geriatric Nurse Practitioner/Physician Team in a Long-Term Care Setting." *HMO Practice* 5 (4): 139–42.

Burl, J. B., and others. 1998. "Geriatric Nurse Practitioners in Long-Term Care: Demonstration of Effectiveness in Managed Care." *Journal of the American Geriatric Society* 46 (4): 506–10.

California HealthCare Foundation. 2001. *Program for Elders in Managed Care* (program material). Oakland, Calif.

Chen, A., and others. 2000. *Best Practices in Coordinated Care*. HCFA 500-95-0048 (04), MPR reference no.: 8534-004. Princeton, N.J.: Mathematica Policy Research.

Coleman, B. 1998. *New Directions for State Long-Term Care Systems*. 2d ed. Washington: AARP Public Policy Institute.

———. 2001. *Consumer-Directed Services for Older People*. Issue brief . Washington: AARP Public Policy Institute.

Coleman, E. A., and others. 1999. "Chronic Care Clinics: A Randomized Controlled Trial of a New Model of Primary Care for Frail Older Adults." *Journal of the American Geriatric Society* 47 (7): 775–83.

Coleman, E. A., and others. 2001. "Reducing Emergency Visits in Older Adults with Chronic Illness: A Randomized, Controlled Trial of Group Visits." *Effective Clinical Practice* 4 (2): 49–57.

Collins, C., and D. Williams. 1999. "Segregation and Mortality: The Deadly Effects of Racism." *Sociological Forum* 14 (3): 495–523.

Conrad, P., and J. W. Schneider. 1992. *Deviance and Medicalization*. Rev. ed. Temple University Press.

DeBusk, R. F., and others. 1994. "A Case-Management System for Coronary Risk Factor Modification after Acute Myocardial Infarction." *Annals of Internal Medicine* 120 (9): 721–29.

Ellrodt, G., and others. 1997. "Evidence-Based Disease Management." *Journal of the American Medical Association* 278 (20): 1687–92.

Eng, C., and others. 1997. "Program of All-Inclusive Care for the Elderly (PACE): An Innovative Model of Integrated Geriatric Care and Financing." *Journal of the American Geriatric Society* 45 (2): 223–32.

Estes, C. L., and E. A. Binney. 1989. "The Biomedicalization of Aging: Dangers and Dilemmas." *Gerontologist* 29 (5): 587–96.

Estes, C. L., M. Casper, and E. A. Binney. 1993. "Empowerment Imperative." In *The Long-Term Care Crisis,* edited by C. L. Estes and J. H. Swan and Associates. Newbury Park, Calif.: Sage Publications.

Estes, C. L., and others. 2001. "The Medicalization and Commodification of Aging and the Privatization and Rationalization of Old Age Policy." In *Social Policy and Aging,* edited by C. L. Estes and Associates. Thousand Oaks, Calif.: Sage Publications.

Fama, T., and P. D. Fox. 1997. "Efforts to Improve Primary Care Delivery to Nursing Home Residents." *Journal of the American Geriatric Society* 45 (5): 627–32.

Farley, D., and others. 1999. "Use of Primary Care Teams by HMOs for Care of Long-Stay Nursing Home Residents." *Journal of the American Geriatric Society* 47 (2): 139–44.

Fireman, B., D. Carpenter, and J. Bartlett. 2000. "Effective Management of Chronic Conditions at Kaiser Permanente, Northern California." Paper presented at the National Academy of Social Insurance Chronic Care Workshop, December 5.

Garrard, J., and others. 1990. "Impact of Geriatric Nurse Practitioners on Nursing-Home Residents' Functional Status, Satisfaction, and Discharge Outcomes." *Medical Care* 28 (3): 271–83.

Harrington, C., M. Lynch, and R. J. Newcomer. 1993. "Medical Services in Social Health Maintenance Organizations." *Gerontologist* 33 (6): 790–800.

Harrington, C., and R. J. Newcomer. 1991. "Social Health Maintenance Organizations' Service Use and Costs, 1985–1989." *Health Care Finance Review* 12 (3): 37–52.

Harrington, C., R. J. Newcomer, and S. Preston. 1993. "A Comparison of S/HMO Disenrollees and Continuing Members." *Inquiry* 30 (4): 429–40.

Irvin, C. V., S. Massey, and T. Dorsey. 1997. "Determinants of Enrollment among Applicants to PACE." *Health Care Finance Review* 19 (2): 135–53.

Joseph, A., and C. Boult. 1998. "Managed Primary Care of Nursing Home Residents." *Journal of the American Geriatric Society* 46 (9): 1152–56.

Kane, R. A., R. L. Kane, and R. C. Ladd. 1998. *The Heart of Long-Term Care.* Oxford University Press.

Kane, R. L., and S. Huck. 2000. "The Implementation of the EverCare Demonstration Project." *Journal of the American Geriatric Society* 48 (2): 218–23.

Kane, R. L., L. H. Illston, and N. A. Miller. 1992. "Qualitative Analysis of the Program of All-Inclusive Care for the Elderly (PACE)." *Gerontologist* 32 (6): 771–80.

Kane, R. L., and others. 1989. "Effects of a Geriatric Nurse Practitioner on Process and Outcome of Nursing Home Care." *American Journal of Public Health* 79 (9): 1271–77.

Kane, R. L., and others. 1997. "S/HMOs, the Second Generation: Building on the Experience of the First Social Health Maintenance Organization Demonstrations." *Journal of the American Geriatric Society* 45 (1): 101–7.

Katon, W., and others. 1995. "Collaborative Management to Achieve Treatment Guidelines: Impact on Depression in Primary Care." *Journal of the American Medical Association* 273 (13): 1026–31.

Knox, D., and L. Mischke. 1999. "Implementing a Congestive Heart Failure Disease Management Program to Decrease Length of Stay and Cost." *Journal of Cardiovascular Nursing* 14 (1): 55–74.

Leveille, S. G., and others. 1998. "Preventing Disability and Managing Chronic Illness in Frail Older Adults: A Randomized Trial of a Community-Based Partnership with Primary Care." *Journal of the American Geriatric Society* 46 (10): 1191–98.

Lorig, K., and others. 1994. *Living a Healthy Life with Chronic Conditions.* Palo Alto, Calif.: Bull Publishing.

Lorig, K. R., and others. 1999. "Evidence Suggesting That a Chronic Disease Self-Management Program Can Improve Health Status While Reducing Hospitalization: A Randomized Trial." *Medical Care* 37 (1): 5–14.

Malone, J. K., D. Chase, and J. Bayard. 1993. "Caring for Nursing Home Residents." *Journal of Health Care Benefits* 2 (3): 51–54.

McCulloch, D. K., and others. 1998. "A Population-Based Approach to Diabetes Management in a Primary Care Setting: Early Results and Lessons Learned." *Effective Clinical Practice* 1 (1): 12–22.

Miller, S. K. 1997. "Impact of a Gerontological Nurse Practitioner on the Nursing Home Elderly in the Acute Care Setting." *AACN Clinical Issues* 8 (4): 609–15.

Mollica, R., and T. Riley. 1997. *Managed Care for Low-Income Elders Dually Eligible for Medicaid and Medicare: A Snapshot of State and Federal Activity.* Portland, Maine: National Academy for State Health Policy.

National Chronic Care Consortium. 2001. *Primary Care for People with Chronic Conditions: Issues and Models. A Technical Assistance Paper of the Robert Wood Johnson Foundation Medicare/Medicaid Integration Program.* University of Maryland Center on Aging.

Newcomer, R., P. Arnsberger, and X. Zhang. 1997. "Case Management, Client Risk Factors, and Service Use." *Health Care Finance Review* 19 (1): 105–20.

Newcomer, R., C. Harrington, and R. Kane. 2000. "Implementing the Second Generation Social Health Maintenance Organization." *Journal of the American Geriatric Society* 48 (7): 829–34.

Newcomer, R., and others. 1995. "Case Mix Controlled Service Use and Expenditures in the Social/Health Maintenance Organization Demonstration." *Journals of Gerontology Series A: Biological Sciences and Medical Sciences* 50A (1): M35–44.

Newcomer, R., and others. 1999. "Effects of the Medicare Alzheimer's Disease Demonstration on Medicare Expenditures." *Health Care Finance Review* 20 (4): 45–65.

Norris, S. L., M. M. Engelgau, and K. M. Narayan. 2001. "Effectiveness of Self-Management Training in Type 2 Diabetes: A Systematic Review of Randomized Controlled Trials." *Diabetes Care* 24 (3): 561–87.

Quinn, J. L., M. Prybylo, and P. Pannone. 1999. "Community Care Management across the Continuum: Study Results from a Medicare Health Maintenance Plan." *Care Management Journal* 1 (4): 223–31.

Rich, M. W. 1999. "Heart Failure Disease Management: A Critical Review." *Journal of Cardiac Failure* 5 (1): 64–75.

Rich, M. W., and others. 1995. "A Multidisciplinary Intervention to Prevent the Readmission of Elderly Patients with Congestive Heart Failure." *New England Journal of Medicine* 333 (18): 1190–95.

Rossiter, L. F., and others. 2000. "The Impact of Disease Management on Outcomes and Cost of Care: A Study of Low-Income Asthma Patients." *Inquiry* 37 (2): 188–202.

Rubin, R. J., K. A. Dietrich, and A. D. Hawk. 1998. "Clinical and Economic Impact of Implementing a Comprehensive Diabetes Management Program in Managed Care." *Journal of Clinical Endocrinology and Metabolism* 83 (8): 2635–42.

Ryan, J. W. 1999. "An Innovative Approach to the Medical Management of the Nursing Home Resident: The EverCare Experience." *Nurse Practitioner Forum* 10 (1): 27–32.

Sadur, C. N., and others. 1999. "Diabetes Management in a Health Maintenance Organization: Efficacy of Care Management Using Cluster Visits." *Diabetes Care* 22 (12): 2011–17.

Schore, J. L., R. S. Brown, and V. A. Cheh. 1999. "Case Management for High-Cost Medicare Beneficiaries." *Health Care Finance Review* 20 (4): 87–101.

Schraeder, C., T. Britt, and P. Shelton. 2000. "Integrated Risk Assessment and Feedback Reporting for Clinical Decision Making in a Medicare Risk Plan." *Journal of Ambulatory Care Management* 23 (4): 40–47.

Shannon, K., and C. Van Reenen. 1998. "PACE (Program of All-Inclusive Care for the Elderly): Innovative Care for the Frail Elderly: Comprehensive Services Enable Most Participants to Remain at Home." *Health Progress* 79 (5): 41–45.

Sikka, R., and others. 1999. "Renal Assessment Practices and the Effect of Nurse Case Management of Health Maintenance Organization Patients with Diabetes." *Diabetes Care* 22 (1): 1–6.

Stuber, J., G. Dallek, and B. Biles. 2001. *National and Local Factors Driving Health Plan Withdrawals from Medicare + Choice: Analyses of Seven Medicare + Choice Markets*. Washington: Commonwealth Fund.

Taylor, C. B., and others. 1997. "The Effect of a Home-Based, Case-Managed, Multifactorial Risk-Reduction Program on Reducing Psychological Distress in Patients with Cardiovascular Disease." *Journal of Cardiopulmonary Rehabilitation* 17 (3): 157–62.

U.S. Department of Health and Human Services. 1998. *Healthy People 2010: Surgeon General's Report on Health Promotion and Disease Prevention*. Washington: Public Health Service.

Wagner, E. H., R. E. Glasgow, and others. 2001. "Quality Improvement in Chronic Illness Care: A Collaborative Approach." *Joint Commission Journal on Quality Improvement* 27 (2): 63–80.

Wagner, E. H., L. C. Grothaus, and others. 2001. "Chronic Care Clinics for Diabetes in Primary Care: A System-Wide Randomized Trial." *Diabetes Care* 24 (4): 695–700.

Wagner, E. H., and others. 1999. "A Survey of Leading Chronic Disease Management Programs: Are They Consistent with the Literature?" *Managed Care Quarterly* 7 (3): 56–66.

Wiener, J. M., and D. G. Stevenson. 1998. "State Policy on Long-Term Care for the Elderly." *Health Affairs (Millwood)* 17 (3): 81–100.

Wiener, J. M., and others. 2001. "What Happened to Long-Term Care in the Health Reform Debate of 1993–1994? Lessons for the Future." *Milbank Quarterly* 79 (2): 207–52.

Wooldridge, J., and others. 2001. *Social Health Maintenance Organizations: Transition into Medicare + Choice.* Contract 500-96-005 (2), submitted to Health Care Financing Administration. Washington.

Yordi, C., and others. 1997. "Caregiver Supports: Outcomes from the Medicare Alzheimer's Disease Demonstration." *Health Care Finance Review* 19 (2): 97–117.

Zimmerman, Y. A., D. Pemberton, and L. Thomas. 1998. *Evaluation of the Program of All-Inclusive Care for the Elderly (PACE) Demonstration: Factors Contributing to Care Management and Decision Making in the PACE Model.* HCFA Contract 500-96-0003/TO4. Washington: HCFA Office of Strategic Planning.

Commentary on Part Four

Comment by Jennie Chin Hansen

I am heartened by Marty Lynch's observation that the integration of acute and long-term care has been perceived to be reasonably successful in the PACE model (the Program of All-Inclusive Care for the Elderly). We can attribute part of our success to our focus on the patients, as Catherine Hawes observes. At On Lok, the first PACE program—and I think it is true of all the other PACE programs—we try to be sure that we remember our purpose: to deliver the care that frail elderly people need in a manner that makes the most sense.

If I had known more than twenty years ago—or if the founder of On Lok, Marie Louise Ansek, had known thirty years ago—what we would be doing today, I think we would have had our heads examined. To create a simple plan for a senior who has multiple chronic diseases, often including degrees of dementia, in addition to functional needs is a tremendous challenge. In the case of On Lok and the entire PACE program, we said, "Let's create a plan that makes sense for our clients. And let's do it in such a way that they don't have to call up Medicare to find out whether they qualify. Let's not wait until they are hospitalized, and thus covered by Medicare, to care for them." An elderly person, for example, may need nutritional attention because she has difficulty eating, but these services are covered only in the hospital, so she will not get the care she needs until some accident or acute episode puts her there. The present system is, in effect, an iatrogenic system; it causes unnecessary pain and suffering to clients; and it is expensive. At On Lok, we try never to forget whom we are serving.

Five Core Principles of the PACE Model

By statute, the PACE model operates under five principles. These principles are listed in the legislation, passed in 1997, that created the program. The first

175

is that we focus exclusively on the frail population. The second is that we focus on comprehensive services across the spectrum, from hospital care, nursing care, and medications to home-care services, day programs, and transportation. The individuals we serve have this whole range of comprehensive services.

The third principle is that we use an interdisciplinary team. Bruce Vladeck notes that the elderly need a whole range of professionals. Our program employs a full range of staff, from geriatricians to home-care staff. We have cardiologists and neurologists, along with whole hospitals, on contract. The fourth defining principle is our form of reimbursement: we blend the inevitable major sources of funding—Medicare and Medicaid. Finally, our fifth principle is that we are a capitated system, meaning we assume financial risk for the care of our enrollees.

Profile of PACE Participants

Who is the typical PACE enrollee? The average age is 82. Participants have seven to nine concomitant medical conditions and a range of degrees of cognitive loss and dementia from 60 to 65 percent. Half of our enrollees are incontinent of their bowel and bladder. Most have functional dependencies with regard to at least three activities of daily living. On average, our patients are on five medications a day.

Growth of PACE

Why has PACE not grown more quickly? Policymakers, state leaders, and major planners are looking for the big solution; the reality, however, is that the people we serve need customized care. Given that our population is frail, our enrollees are much more similar to nursing-home populations—which average about a hundred beds each—than Kaiser Permanente's population. So comparing the Kaiser program, with an enrollment of 13 million, and On Lok in San Francisco, with nine hundred enrollees, is like comparing apples and oranges.

A typical nursing-home staffing ratio, for example, is 1.1 staff to one resident. This explains why care in a nursing home is so expensive. In On Lok, we have about sixty-seven staff for every hundred residents. Like the nursing home, we are staff-intensive, care-intensive, and therefore expensive.

It is difficult to get providers to switch gears from the linear silos they face in their professional fields—to use a metaphor that has been associated with Medicare and Medicaid. We face some of the same problems as those Bruce Fireman ascribes to Kaiser, especially getting our providers to work together as a team. Finding a common language for the diverse professionals caring for each patient is a challenge.

I often compare our health-care teams to football teams. The doctor is usually the quarterback, but sometimes the ball is passed to one of the other players, and someone else has a chance to make the goal. A good team works together to make that happen. For providers to change their usual practice and accept this kind of play takes a lot of de-conditioning. I used to ask team members as they joined us to leave their guns at the door.

Moreover, the capital needs of developing our program are still quite large. In addition to the start-up costs, we need to secure a continuing operating budget. In a risk-adjusted compensated system such as ours, with a high degree of complexity, capitalization, changing systems, and risk taking, it is crucial that we stay ahead of our income flow.

Owing to the need to manage and keep all the balls in the air at the same time, then, in addition to start-up challenges, a PACE program may not be easy to set up—as health-care systems are beginning to realize. Simply put, it is extremely hard to alter the regular financing system in the care of very frail elders. Little did we know, when we started, that we were talking about reformatting the Medicare and Medicaid financing and delivery systems—that we would have them working as a team to ensure an effective response to the complex medical, cognitive, and functional needs of this population.

These are some of the challenges that the PACE program has encountered, but there are now twenty-five PACE programs serving dual eligibles operating around the country. Fourteen others are under Medicaid, and probably another half dozen are in planning stages. So despite these challenges, there is some opportunity. Is PACE the panacea? The answer is no. It was never intended to be solve all the problems in long-term care, but it is a model of care service delivery and financing that does work in communities and from which much can be learned.

Comment by Bruce C. Vladeck

Although I sometimes think that the only accomplishment in long-term care over the past thirty years has been that I am that much closer to needing the care, I know that we have made some progress and learned some lessons. Most impressive to me was the consistency of the lessons learned across all of the presentations of the panel.

The first lesson is one we have to keep relearning: when we talk about very frail old people with significant chronic illness, doctors really matter. The more we move away from "the medical model" of service provision, the more important the relationship between the service delivery organization and the physician becomes. The clients, by definition, have serious, complicated medical problems, which create all or part of the need for the services that we think of as nonmedical. The interaction between the medical problems, the health problems of patients and clients, and the other services is constant and critical.

To cast the same point in the negative, everyone who has ever worked in a nursing home or a community-based long-term-care program knows that the worst possible thing that can happen to a client, no matter how well she has been taken care of, is hospitalization, in the hands of a physician who has no relationship with the program. In the absence of this relationship, months of hard work can be undone remarkably fast. To be sure, given the way the health-care system is constituted in most communities, figuring out the right form of relationship with physicians can be tricky, but without it, service programs for the frail elderly are never going to get terribly far.

The second lesson is that multidisciplinary teamwork is really essential for good care of chronically ill, frail people over any period of time. Such teamwork is rare and hard to achieve. In the training of health-care profession-als, particularly physicians and nurses, one of the things that is emphasized strongly is personal accountability for the well-being of the patient. Nurses and physicians are taught a degree of thoroughness and conscientiousness associ-ated with the fulfillment of their professional role, demanding that they take responsibility for their professional practice. This training makes it difficult to turn a group of professionals into a team.

The third lesson is one that many participants have noted in a number of different ways through individual cases. I offer a systematic generalization: to oversimplify (only slightly), after thousands of studies, millions of miles of data tapes (when we still had tapes), and lots of analyses, the bottom line is that, on average, it is clear that nothing ever saves money. I was administrator of the Health Care Financing Administration for 1,571 days, and on every one of them at least one person said to me, "If you do X or Y, it will save Medicare a lot of money." So I had to come up with some kind of stock response, and the one I finally arrived at was, "Nothing ever saves Medicare any money." There were always plenty of empirical cases I could adduce to support that assertion.

In long-term care, there are at least three reasons why nothing ever saves money. At the root of each is a significant policy question that poses dilemmas that may in some way be irresoluble. First, we do not have any comprehensive way of accounting for all the costs associated with the lives of our clients and their families and caregivers. So for a number of years, we kept making the mistake of comparing the cost of service delivery to people living in their homes, who were paying for their food and rent out of their own pockets, with the total costs of caring for people in institutions—which, of course, included room and board. Home care obviously looked cheaper.

We have spent a considerable amount of time reinforcing the confusion about different "levels of care" and believing that each level would have its own specific costs, regardless of the services delivered to the people within them. Of course, we are always making policy on the basis of cost to a particular payer, so if something is cheaper for Medicare, it quite possibly is more expensive for Medicaid. Medicare does not worry as much because the federal government is only paying 54 cents on the Medicaid dollar.

Second, other than by constraining the supply of nursing-home beds in certain markets or by limiting total enrollment in home- and community-based waiver programs, we have never figured out a way to control the volume of services we are going to provide, and we have never figured out a set of definitions that make any clinical, logical, and administrative sense of the eligibility rules. Need for service is a complicated, fuzzy issue: people's characteristics are often ambiguous, and their needs change continually. Part of this is the so-called woodwork effect; that is, if the amount of long-term care provided is increased without limits being imposed on its capacity, needy clients will "come out of the woodwork," and demand will be greater than anticipated. Another part is the political and administrative difficulty of enforcing selective admissions policies based solely or primarily on risk screening. Given the pressures, eligibility barriers tend to erode quickly.

Finally, of course, the great dirty secret of the Medicare program that has become increasingly apparent in recent years is that it is the only health insurer in the United States that keeps all of its beneficiaries until they die. So if Medicare does a really good job and keeps its beneficiaries living longer, that is a wash, at best, from the point of view of the Medicare trust funds. The better Medicare does in managing potentially fatal chronic illnesses like congestive heart failure, the less savings it achieves from premature mortality of beneficiaries with heart failure.

On the other hand, I think the data are clear that, if we do a better job of providing care, whether in comprehensive community-based services through a PACE program or through a somewhat less comprehensive set of services supported by some Medicaid home- and community-based waivers, or through better clinical services revolving around disease, we do measurably improve the quality of care. So maybe we would all be better off if we put some of the cost arguments aside, at least while trying to think of how to design better service delivery systems. I recommend we try first to figure out what quality care is and then figure out how to pay for it in a way that is politically acceptable.

As a final generalization, I would suggest that we need to stop beating ourselves over the head about the rate of progress. Long-term care is really hard to provide. Providing regular medical care to a healthy population is quite simple by comparison. Providing social services unrelated to people's illnesses is also relatively simple. By definition, long-term-care patients are very sick; their problems are clinically and physiologically complicated; they have multiple diagnoses that interact in all sorts of weird ways; they are disproportionately poor and therefore without a lot of other resources immediately available to them or to their families or the households in which they live. The problems for which we are trying to help them exhibit lots of ambiguity.

In passing, let me note that it is also impossible to deal with chronically ill patients over time without recognizing the importance of informal caregivers. Chronic illness happens not just to individuals but to their families, as well. Yet Medicare and Medicaid provide entitlements to individuals, not to families.

So I do think we have to be a little bit more clearheaded about evaluating ourselves and our own performance. We have made significant progress in at least some areas. We probably have not saved a nickel in the process, and we are not going to as we go forward. But if we can figure out how to engage doctors better, how to develop and maintain real multidisciplinary teams, how to define the elements of care that make for high quality, I think we can continue to make things better, one marginal step at a time.

PART FIVE

Visions for the Future:
How Might We Meet Tomorrow's Needs for Chronic and Long-Term Care?

14

Private Long-Term-Care Solutions: The Government as Employer

John Cutler

T HE HISTORY OF THE Federal Long Term Care Insurance Program begins with the demise of President Bill Clinton's health-care reform effort. With Congress and the American people signaling problems for large social insurance fixes in health care, the administration turned elsewhere for solutions to these problems after the 1996 election.

In 1998 and 1999 the administration presented a small set of incremental but compatible solutions across a number of areas involving long-term care. One proposed a caregiver tax credit of up to $1,000 (later raised to $3,000). Another was an initiative for the Administration on Aging to provide grants to the states for innovative caregiver training and related programs. A third initiative was an education campaign by Medicare encouraging citizens to look elsewhere than Medicare (and Medicaid) for solutions to their long-term-care needs. A fourth was to have the federal government, acting as employer, provide long-term-care insurance to its employees.

All were fairly well received on a bipartisan basis, although the concern over the cost of some of the items (especially the caregiver tax credit) was problematic. Indeed, ultimately, all but the caregiver tax credit passed. Perhaps most reflective of the bipartisanship was what became known as the Federal Long Term Care Insurance Program.

The Long-Term Care Security Act (P.L. 106-265) passed in the summer of 2000 and was signed into law on September 19, 2000. It authorized the U.S. Office of Personnel Management (OPM) to contract for a long-term-care insurance program. The OPM expects that, like the health and life insurance programs it administers, the Federal Long Term Care Insurance Program will become the largest employer-sponsored long-term-care insurance program in the nation.

Currently, the largest employer-sponsored program is the CalPERS (California Public Employees' Retirement System) Long-Term Care Pro-

184 JOHN CUTLER

gram.[1] That program's success derives from a competitive product (in terms of both price and features), an extensive and sustained awareness and education campaign, and the size of the eligible population. The federal program hopes to incorporate into its marketing campaign these key elements of success— building agency support, maintaining a competitive product, and emphasizing the continued importance of education and reenrollment activities.

One of the real advantages of the Federal Long Term Care Insurance Program is that it is an employer-sponsored product that the OPM considers to be an important part of the government's overall compensation package. This means the policy must be competitive with the best policies offered by other employers.

Coverage will be available (with underwriting) to federal employees and annuitants as well as active and retired members of the uniformed services. Also covered are "qualified relatives" of active workers and military personnel. This includes spouses, adult children, parents, and parents-in-law. The OPM may make coverage available to additional groups (for example, former spouses and domestic partners) by regulation. Interestingly enough, congressional input here added some key features. Access of the military was important to Representative Connie Morella (R-Md.), while provision for spouses to have equal or equivalent underwriting was important to Representative Henry Waxman (D-Calif.). Both these concepts were added to the bill during the debate on its passage.

The law states that coverage must become effective not later than October 2002, but the OPM was easily able to beat that deadline. An early enrollment period was established from March 25 to May 15, 2002. Open season started July 1 and extended through December 31, 2002.

The opportunity for early enrollment was another congressional concept. Senator Bob Graham (D-Fla.), among others, suggested that there was no reason to wait for development of the full education effort for many individuals, who already knew about the risk of needing long-term-care services and were anxious to buy insurance. Open season, though, is more along the lines of what the OPM had been told by carriers and consumers was important for a successful offering. The importance of educating the work force and other

---

1. Perhaps as many as 5 million people are eligible for the CalPERS program, compared with the federal program's reach of 20 million. CalPERS has about 160,000 enrollees after eight years. In both cases the total includes a significant proportion of people with whom the sponsor has no direct contact—and to whom, therefore, the sponsor cannot market—and many eligibles who have a weak relationship with the group (for example, parents of enrollees) and are therefore unlikely to buy.

eligibles about long-term-care risks and the value of having insurance is considered paramount in terms of a successful employer offering. This includes educating people about the fact that Medicare, Medicaid, employer-provided health insurance, and other insurance products are not going to cover this problem or will not do so in the best way. The insurers plan literally thousands of meetings, coverage on TV and radio in some markets, direct mail to some populations, and other outreach efforts.

The OPM obtained broad input from the insurance industry, experts and actuaries, consumer and aging groups, and other stakeholders such as federal retiree groups like the National Association of Retired Federal Employees and the Retired Officers Association. This input helped define the product design released by the _____ _____ in the spring of 2001. Ultimately, two c _____ ntract. (The law provide _____ consortium" arrangem _____ carrier could carry out _____ all the eligible member _____

One such cc _____ ife. The other was led by _____ r and the Long Term Ca _____ reat deal of experience i _____ mployers because they h _____ ate plans.

Ultimately, _____ icock and MetLife as th _____ under the Federal Long _____ formed a joint venture _____ lusively to administering _____ er because of the strengu. _____ of the two together to meet the needs of the OPM through that n.... .....

[Handwritten note: About OPM, seems to work well — comparable rates]

What was interesting in the Request for Proposal process and final negotiations was that the design of the insurance would look very much like what is currently available on the individual market sold through insurers and agents. (Eighty percent of sales in the United States are through individual agents.) However, it is expected that (like most employer-provided group plans) the coverage will be provided with less underwriting and form completion and at a discounted rate. How much of a discount? The OPM had hoped for 15 to 20 percent below a comparable product that might be sold by an agent—the theory being that if agent compensation added roughly 10 percent and the federal program had other economies of scale, it would be possible to beat the competition by about that much.

What was not adequately taken into account was that "comparability" is almost impossible to determine. For example, active employees and their spouses have extremely abbreviated underwriting. This makes it difficult for consumers to examine their options in an apples-to-apples kind of comparison. Yet it definitely has an impact on premium costs. Similarly, the OPM's inclusion of international coverage, informal caregiving, independent third-party review in the event of a claims dispute, and other features unique to the program all have value that does not show up in a premium comparison.

In this regard, the OPM has stated that though it "may not be able to beat the most deeply discounted premiums in the private market, we think we will be able to offer better value. That means better value in terms of premium stability and because, as an employer-sponsor, we will ensure that the policy evolves as the provision of long-term care services changes in the future. The policy will be contemporary when purchased and thirty or more years later when it is needed."[2] The experiences of other groups, such as CalPERS and AARP, show that such expectations are valid, as each has kept its coverage current through expansions in benefits without any increase in rates.

By statute, there will be no government contribution to the premium. The absence of a subsidy puts the product on a par with individual insurance, which, of course, has no subsidy. It does distinguish it, however, from other federal employee benefits. In fact, the plan that covers health insurance for the civilian work force, the Federal Employees Health Benefit Program, not only includes a large subsidy of 80 to 90 percent of premium costs; coverage is issued on a guaranteed basis, as well. (Unlike health insurance, however, long-term-care insurance is guaranteed renewable and fully portable.)

When the dust settled, the OPM's specific product design was basically a comprehensive policy covering everything from home care to nursing homes. It was set up as an indemnity product as opposed to the disability model (such as those used by Aetna and UNUM). A person's daily benefit amount multiplied by the number of years of coverage creates a "pool of money" that is available to draw upon if the need for care is triggered. Expenses incurred are paid up to the daily benefit maximum the insured selects.

It should be mentioned that Congress required that the policy be "tax qualified." Under the Health Insurance Portability and Accountability Act (HIPAA) of 1996, insurance coverage is triggered if a person needs help with at least two of six activities of daily living (ADLs) for at least ninety days or has

2. Remarks by Kay Coles James, director of the U.S. Office of Personnel Management, press conference, July 1, 2002.

a severe cognitive impairment. The statute requires that any policy the OPM puts into place meet Internal Revenue Service qualification requirements and be compliant with HIPAA tax-qualification requirements.

For the most part, the HIPAA also requires that the OPM follow the full standards of the National Association of Insurance Commissioners (NAIC). However, the OPM can deviate from individual market standards in two ways. First, the law allows the OPM to preempt state long-term-care insurance laws. This is important for a federal program seeking to provide uniform coverage across its work force and to establish the supremacy of the federal government over its own operations (something that is true across all federal activities, going well beyond insurance).

Second, the HIPAA allows the policyholder to exercise some rights. In the group offering, the employer is the policyholder and the employee is a certificate holder. When the employer is the policyholder, however, as is the case with a federal insurance program, it may mean that an employee sees a different set of features in a group offering than he or she would in the individual market. For example, many employers offer only one kind of inflation protection, usually reduce the choices relating to daily benefit amount and length of coverage, and may not bother to offer facility-only coverage. The OPM chose to exercise its policyholder rights only once and in a way that distinguishes its product from individual products that comply with the NAIC. That was on the issue of the offer of nonforfeiture.[3]

Because the OPM believed there would be little value in extending the offer to prospective purchasers, it employed two other tools of the NAIC to provide some protection to its insureds. One is that it follows a companion provision called contingent nonforfeiture. This is a protection consumers do not have to choose; it springs into action if the insurer takes a rate increase over a certain amount that forces insureds to let their policies lapse because they cannot or do not wish to pay the higher premium. The other benefit, which is often not spelled out by insurers, is the right to "downgrade" a policy, that is, to reduce the amount of coverage so that the premium is reduced.

---

3. Nonforfeiture is essentially insurance in case of lapse, that is, insurance on insurance. A person who allows the policy to lapse and has a nonforfeiture benefit would retain some value. Typically, this is not monetary. Instead, it is some form of reduced coverage that will continue to exist even without further premium payments. This amount is actuarially related to the value of premiums already paid by that person. A discussion of how the NAIC came to develop the requirement of such an offer is too extensive for the scope of this paper; for our purposes, suffice it to say that almost no one takes this offer. (It is rather expensive and provides only a limited amount of coverage upon lapse.)

The Federal Long Term Care Insurance Program followed the NAIC rate stabilization rules in setting premiums. The OPM elected not to make the product noncancelable, meaning a guarantee that there will never be a rate increase. To do that would have required a significant additional surcharge to the premium. Yet in reality rate increases in the employer market are rare, and neither John Hancock nor MetLife has ever raised rates on any of their existing employer business policies.

One unique feature, also added during the congressional passage, was third-party review of claims disputes. Although it is a standard fixture in health insurance, it is almost unheard of in long-term-care insurance. However, the OPM is required to establish a system that provides an insured who has a disagreement with a claims decision made by the insurers the right to an independent third-party review. (The decision to insure is not subject to third-party review; it is solely at the insurers' discretion.)

Another interesting component of the OPM offering was the thought that went into coverage for those who could not be insured. Because everyone undergoes some form of health screening (underwriting) before becoming insured, some will be turned down for coverage. (However, the screening for active employees consists of only seven questions, and for their spouses only nine, the additional two serving as surrogates for determining whether the spouse is as healthy as someone actively working.) For some people who are refused coverage, there will be nonstandard insurance that is more limited, and higher premiums will reflect the higher risk. For all others who are refused, the OPM offers a "service package" that is not insurance. The service package includes access to care coordination and discounts for health-care products and services. Individuals decide whether or not they want to purchase this service package.

At this early writing there is every reason to think the program is off to a good start. However, even a fabulously successful offering does not come close to covering the long-term-care risks that Americans face. Thus as important as this is from an insurance perspective, the real public policy story still lies in the future.

Appendix 14A: The Federal Long Term Care Insurance Program

The Federal Long Term Care Insurance Program includes the following features:

—comprehensive coverage, including reimbursement for care in a nursing home, care in an assisted-living facility, formal and informal care in the home, hospice care, and respite services

—facilities-only coverage

—choice of a daily benefit amount, in various multiples[4]

—choice of a length of benefit payment: three years, five years, or lifetime

—choice of waiting period: thirty or ninety days[5]

—choice of inflation protection options: automatic compound inflation (at 5 percent a year) or future purchase option (following the consumer price index's medical index)

—two ways to trigger benefit: by being certified as needing substantial assistance with at least two of six activities of daily living, those needs expected to last at least ninety days; or by being severely cognitively impaired, such as by Alzheimer's disease

—for some active employees or their spouses who do not pass the underwriting (depending on their condition), an alternative insurance offering (which essentially covers only facility care); for all individuals who fail to pass underwriting, a service package offering, which includes access to care coordination and discounts

Eligible Groups (the Federal Family)

The estimate for the core of the "federal family" (employees, retirees, and their spouses) eligible for coverage is around 8 million, but the total eligible pool could approach or exceed 20 million people. As specified in the law, those eligible to apply for the insurance include

—federal employees (including postal employees and members of the uniformed services and some others, such as Tennessee Valley Authority employees but not employees of the District of Columbia government)

—annuitants (including retired members of the uniformed services and survivors of deceased federal employees or federal annuitants receiving a survivor annuity, as well as some others)

4. The choice can also be weekly if a comprehensive plan is selected.

5. The waiting period counts days the insured pays for covered services out-of-pocket or through other insurance. It does not count calendar days. The waiting period needs to be satisfied only once over the lifetime of the policy.

—qualifying relatives: spouses of employees and annuitants (including survivors of deceased members or retired members of the uniformed services receiving survivor annuities), adult children of employees and annuitants (at least eighteen years old, including adopted children and stepchildren), and parents, parents-in-law, and step-parents of employees (but not of annuitants)

The law gives the OPM authority to issue regulations to cover other qualified relatives. This might occur in 2003.

Underwriting

Underwriting of insured employees falls under one of two categories. All applicants other than active federal employees, members of the uniformed services, and their spouses will be subject to full underwriting. This means that they will have to answer numerous health-related questions. It may also include a review of medical records or a personal interview (or both). This is the same level of underwriting that those who purchase individual policies in the private market undergo.

Federal employees, members of the uniformed services, and their spouses will be subject to abbreviated underwriting: they will be required to complete a short-form application, which asks fewer health-related questions. Spouses will be asked for some additional information as a substitute for not being actively at work for the government. (For those applying for lifetime coverage, there are some additional questions.)

Contact Information

Two websites have been set up: one by the OPM at www.opm.gov/insure/ltc, the other by Long Term Care Partners at www.ltcfeds.com. A toll-free number has also been set up by the carriers: 1-800-582-3337.

15

The Life Care Annuity: A Better Approach to Financing Long-Term Care and Retirement Income

Mark Warshawsky

THE PROVISION AND financing of long-term care and retirement income pose significant and growing problems, now and projected for the future, for both the public and private sectors. For the public sector, spending by Medicaid and Medicare on various types of long-term care—mainly home health care and nursing-home care—is already large and is projected to grow substantially as costs increase and the population ages. Yet there are real constraints on the budgets of the federal and state governments to finance these increases in spending; tax increases are not a desirable option; and the long-range financial position of the Medicare programs is in deep negative balance. Through various eligibility and spend-down rules and look-back provisions, Medicaid was designed to function as a welfare program to provide health insurance to the poor, and it is not well suited to provide financing for the long-term-care needs of the middle-class retired population. It does not support the values of prudence, saving, and long-range planning.

Regarding retirement income, employer-sponsored pensions are moving away from the provision of guaranteed life-annuity income, on either a mandatory or an optional basis, in a defined-benefit plan. Rather, the trend is toward defined-contribution plans that impose less structure on the disposition of assets at retirement. At the same time there are serious policy discussions about Social Security personalization—that is, giving people the option to move some of their payroll taxes into individual accounts. These trends and discussions, which could lead to increased risk exposure arising from uncertainty about the length of life, highlight the importance of enhancing the

Some of the work underlying this paper was done while the author was a visiting research scholar at the National Bureau of Economic Research in New York City. The paper reflects prior academic work by the author and does not reflect an official position of the current administration.

attractiveness of a voluntary life-annuity option in various types of retirement plans.

Yet an appropriate and often optimal way of responding to the financial security needs of most households in the face of uncertainty—insurance plans and programs provided and financed through the private sector—also currently exhibits some problems. Strict underwriting excludes a significant percentage of the retired population, mainly those in relatively poor health, from coverage by private long-term-care insurance. Although long-term-care insurance benefits in private insurance policies have improved greatly over the past decade, while premium rates have been stable or declined slightly, further improvements, especially in terms of flexibility, would be desirable. The existence of long-term-care benefits in the Medicaid and Medicare programs would tend to discourage the use of private long-term-care insurance by many households. Indeed, the current Medicaid structure may instead encourage the transfer of some financial assets just before or at entrance into a nursing home to secure nursing-home care paid by Medicare when the three-year look-back period of the spend-down rules ends. Moreover, a recent survey conducted by the North Carolina State Department of Health and Human Services indicates that most states had collected very little from estate recovery efforts—only about 0.26 percent of Medicaid expenditures.[1] This level of effort may indicate that Medicaid as currently designed and administered will cover long-term-care expenses adequately for middle-class households with active interests in leaving assets to heirs.

Finally, the natural operation of adverse selection in voluntary annuity markets continues to cause the price of immediate life annuities to be higher than may be attractive to many retired households of average or below-average expected longevity. (The immediate life annuity is a simple insurance product whereby a sum of money is paid in return for payment by the insurance company or plan sponsor of periodic benefits for the remainder of the annuitant's life.) This is true even as stable or declining interest rates and declining expected equity market returns have made annuities relatively more attractive as an investment class.

There are many possible solutions to these problems, and some are currently being tried or proposed. For the past six years, I have been suggesting one possible private sector solution that attempts to deal with all of the problems simultaneously: the integration of long-term-care insurance benefits with the life annuity. Indeed, in prior empirical research, my coinvestigators, Chris Murtaugh and Brenda Spillman, and I have shown that the life expectancy of

1. Beth Kidder and Susan Harmuth, North Carolina Department of Health and Human Services, 1998. Survey summary at 222.ltclink.net/reference/ref_medicaid_recovery.html.

purchasers of an integrated product would be less than that of voluntary purchasers of immediate life annuities. We have also shown that, with minimal underwriting, the cost of the integrated product would be less than the sum of the cost of two products sold separately. Moreover, the population attracted to the integrated product would be significantly larger than the group of persons who can and likely will purchase the life annuity and long-term care insurance separately; in particular, this expanded population will include most of those denied, through underwriting, access to coverage by long-term-care insurance.[2]

This paper advocates a private sector solution—an integrated insurance product that I call the life care annuity—to the public and private sector problems outlined above. This is consistent with a political philosophy emphasizing individual responsibility and personal choice as well as a concern to minimize the size of government programs. At the same time, this paper tentatively explores those aspects of government policy that currently discourage, or at least fail to encourage, the actual implementation of the integration idea presented here.

Long-Term-Care Insurance

Although the need for long-term care may be thought to be a natural result of the aging process affecting everyone equally (and therefore best funded through retirement saving), it actually is a risk fairly well suited to insurance coverage. In particular, almost half of the retired population will have little or no need for long-term care, and for many others, the need will be of short duration or of relatively little additional cost. For a significant segment of the population, however—knowable in advance, in a probabilistic sense, through actuarial and other empirical studies—the need for care will be of lengthy duration and substantial additional cost. Hence long-term care may be considered an insurable contingency.

Insurance companies have been selling long-term-care insurance policies for the past three decades, although it is only in the past ten years or so that sales have increased significantly. The market seems to be competitive, as more than a hundred companies actively issue and market policies. As has been noted above, benefits in the insurance contracts have improved steadily and significantly, and premium rates have been stable or declining, according to industry statistics, as insurance companies have gained confidence in their knowledge of the relevant risks based on experience and study. So, in terms of the premium-to-coverage ratio, costs of this insurance have declined over time.

2. For the empirical evidence, see Murtaugh, Spillman, and Warshawsky (2001).

There is also a plethora of choices, both among insurance companies and even within a single policy series offered by a particular company, allowing for a tailoring of coverage to specific individual needs and preferences.

The recent growth in the market for long-term-care insurance is all the more remarkable given current government policy in this area. In a theoretical analysis, Mark Pauly has shown that purchase of private long-term-care insurance is nonrational in the presence of Medicaid unless the household has a strong preference for choice in the type and location of the care its members might receive.[3] Of course, the purchase of private long-term-care insurance reduces reliance on public sector programs and encourages rational long-range planning and saving by households. The current tax treatment of long-term-care insurance premiums and benefits for "qualified" policies reflecting certain legal standards for benefit provisions is modestly encouraging, although there are substantial savings to state and federal governments in reduced Medicaid spending.

Long-term-care insurance also currently suffers from some inherent problems. The most significant one is that, at current modal ages of purchase, around retirement, about a quarter of the relevant (aged) population would be rejected by insurance companies from buying long-term-care insurance under current underwriting criteria. Of course, purchase of insurance at a younger age largely avoids the underwriting problem but at the cost of freezing in place for a potentially lengthy stretch of time a certain mode of care reflected in the type of benefits provided in the policy purchased. Youthful purchase also increases risk arising from uncertainty about the continuity of the issuing insurer. Considering that, for example, a long-term-care insurance policy purchased at the age of 55—a typical early retirement age—could be in force for more than forty years, these risk factors can become quite significant as the household ages. Another disadvantage is that most current policies employ indemnity or reimbursement of cost approaches, which are somewhat inflexible, not allowing for free choice in modes of treatment and care. Moreover, long-term-care insurance policyholders bear some added risk arising from the allowance by state regulations for insurers to increase premiums on a class of policies issued. (Actual utilization of this permission, however, has not been widespread.)

All of these disadvantages have good reasons grounded in conservative business practices and insurance regulations—the protection of the insurance company and its customers. Nevertheless, they come at a price in risk and flexibility for the consumer, which, in turn, suggests the consideration of alternative insurance policy designs in the private sector. Finally, experience

3. See Pauly (1990).

has been that some policyholders allow their long-term-care insurance policies to lapse, even after several years of premium payments, and are therefore uninsured precisely at the older ages when insurance coverage is most needed. This problem could be circumvented through better product design, as well.

The Life Annuity

The life-annuity insurance product serves an essential purpose: to spread a stock of resources over the lifetime of an individual or a couple, regardless of how long that may be. The issuing insurance company does this by pooling many individuals' resources together and paying those individuals who live beyond the average life expectancy of the insured group with assets remaining from individuals who died before the average life expectancy. Because few know when they are going to die, individuals with similar expectations of longevity will be willing to enter a risk pool together to insure against two adverse outcomes: running out of money and needing to husband resources, thereby cheating themselves of a comfortable life-style. The insurance company issuing the annuities is able to take the mortality risk it is assuming because mortality statistics for the general population and various groups are available and generally accurate, and trends in mortality are slow to change and seem to be largely predictable.

Successive empirical studies have shown that the money's worth of single-premium immediate annuities sold in the private market has improved significantly in recent years as interest rates have declined and stabilized.[4] In addition, many varieties of immediate annuities are available, including fixed, increasing, and variable annuities, which allow households to choose the risk profile for income payments with which they will be most comfortable. Many different payment structures are also available, such as life with period certain and joint-and-survivor, which allow for a choice among survivorship rights and thus address, in a limited fashion, a bequest motive. Life annuities are found in Social Security, qualified retirement plans, after-tax investment vehicles such as deferred annuities, and even as reverse annuity mortgages, whereby housing equity is unlocked for a household while continued residence in the original residence and a steady income for life are ensured.

Yet annuities also suffer from at least two disadvantages. First, life annuities sold in a voluntary market may fail to attract those individuals who are in poor health or who otherwise perceive themselves to have a lower-than-average life expectancy; that is, life annuities can experience adverse selection of mortality

---

4. Many of these published articles are collected in Brown and others (2001).

risks. Because short-lived people do not enter the risk pool, the issuing insurance company must set the price of the life annuity to reflect its expectation of the equilibrium life expectancy of the purchasing group, which turns out to be higher than that of the general population. Unless they can form risk pools of their own, individuals with shortened life expectancies do not purchase life annuities and may be left exposed to whatever lifetime uncertainty remains for them (even for the sick, length of life is rarely known for certain in advance). Individuals with longer life expectancies are happy to purchase the life annuities available in the market but obviously would be happier still if their risk pool were expanded to include a wider range of people.

Second, life annuities are illiquid. This illiquidity is an essential design feature because without it, insurance companies would be dynamically subject to adverse selection. That is, individuals who purchased immediate annuities with the expectation that their lifetimes would be at least "average" for the group, but who after a period of time discovered that their lifetimes were likely to be short, would want to cash in their annuities at that time if they were allowed to do so. The issuing insurance company, of course, to protect its mortality assumptions in pricing the contracts, does not allow cash dissolution of its immediate-annuity contracts. The resulting illiquidity can pose a problem, however, for the household that has no other assets when an emergency demanding extra resources arises. Obviously there are many types of emergencies, but for the elderly these cash needs are often health related, including long-term-care needs, as the relevant insurances covering these types of emergencies are either incomplete, unavailable, or have not been purchased.

"Do-It-Yourself" Combination of Products

As mentioned above, I am suggesting as an alternative to current products an integrated insurance product providing both life-annuity and long-term-care benefits in the belief that it will mitigate many of the problems with current products and will better address the current needs of households and public policy. To evaluate such an approach, it is important first to have a more detailed description of the long-term-care insurance and life-annuity products that are currently available in the market, including their premium costs and how they might be combined in a "do-it-yourself" way. What does a long-term-care insurance policy with certain specified benefit features cost a 65-year-old individual? What does a single-premium immediate annuity cost a 65-year-old individual? If the two products are combined, what are the net costs and benefits? A simple exercise was conducted at the end of December 2001, using insurance products marketed directly over the Internet, to find answers to these questions.

One large senior citizens' organization markets, on its website, a long-term-care insurance policy issued by a large insurer. In some respects, the policy design is ahead of the rest of the industry—in particular, in including a small informal home-care benefit—but it is therefore difficult to know whether the cost of the policy is competitive. Nevertheless, because this policy is readily available to everyone and the organizations involved have good reputations, we chose it as the basis of our analysis.

As in most policies, the insured here is eligible for benefits if he or she is impaired in two of six activities of daily living (ADLs) or is cognitively impaired. Unlimited duration of coverage was chosen, based on the view that, abstracting from Medicaid, a rational person would especially want to cover his or her greatest and most expensive risks, which are contained in the long tail of the long-term-care need distribution. We selected a benefit of $4,200 a month in maximum reimbursement for nursing-home care, which would cover the current cost of a nursing-home stay in most parts of the country, excluding a few urban areas. The home- and adult-care benefit was put at 50 percent of the nursing-home benefit. As mentioned above, this particular policy pays for informal home care at 25 percent of the nursing-home benefit; unlike the other benefits in the policy, this benefit is not reimbursement for actual expenses incurred. The policy is nonforfeitable and offers a premium waiver in the event the insured becomes impaired. This particular policy features a short standard waiting period for benefits—thirty days. To lower the quoted premium, however, and to better reflect most households' likely risk preferences, the waiting period was adjusted to ninety days. The premium for the adjusted policy was calculated to be $165 a month, purchased at age 65, based on a ratio of quoted premiums using another prominent insurance company's almost identical direct-marketed policy with thirty-day and ninety-day waiting periods.

The second half of the combination strategy is a single-premium immediate life annuity, with a ten-year guarantee period (that is, it pays benefits for at least ten years), issued by a AAA-rated commercial insurance company that sells exclusively over the Internet. Because this company changes its rates as often as daily, it presumably is competitive in the life-annuity market. Premiums for individual policies paying $1,165 a month were sought on the website for a 65-year-old man and woman and were combined in equal proportions to produce a gender-neutral rate. The cost of this annuity was $171,511 at the end of December 2001.

By buying the long-term-care insurance policy described above, then, for a monthly premium of $165 and a single-premium immediate annuity paying $1,165 monthly at a cost of $171,511, the insured gets, net before taxes, $1,000 in monthly income for life while he or she is in good health. If the insured has a disability requiring home care, he or she will get approximately $3,000 a month for life. If the insured becomes disabled and has to go into a nursing home, he or she will get more than $5,000 a month for as long as the insured is disabled, including up to $4,000 to pay for nursing-home care. This is a nice combination, covering both the risk of having a long life and the risk of needing long-term care.[5]

If the immediate life annuity were purchased using after-tax money, regular payments would be taxed according to the so-called exclusion ratio, which is a largely fair approach that taxes only interest earnings and not the return of principal. If the immediate life annuity were purchased using qualified retirement plan assets, the entire stream of regular payments would be subject to income taxation. Assuming that the long-term-care insurance policy were "qualified," periodic premiums would be deductible, subject to limits dependent on the age of purchase and to an overall restriction that noninsured allowable health and other expenses, including policy premiums, exceed 7.5 percent of adjusted gross income. Payments from the long-term-care policy whose design meets the requirements of the tax law and regulations are not taxable.

What are the disadvantages of this combination of products? First, applicants would still have to undergo health screening to secure underwriting for the long-term-care insurance policy, so many would be turned down. Another disadvantage is that this combination includes a fairly traditional long-term-care insurance policy, and so it largely covers reimbursement only for expenses incurred. If the insured were to decide, for example, to have his or her care provided by a relative or close friend in exchange for a payment, this policy would pay only a nominal amount. Furthermore, there is the possibility that the insurance company could increase long-term-care premiums for a class of insureds, although the particular insurance company issuing the policy we are using apparently has never increased premiums. There is the risk that the individual might allow his or her long-term-care insurance policy to lapse. Moreover, in a voluntary single-premium immediate annuity, the premium rate is relatively high because of adverse selection—that is, because of a tendency for only people in the best, or at least good, health to buy it.

The Integrated Approach

The life care annuity—or as I have also called it, more technically, the single-premium immediate disability escalating annuity—is an integration of the life annuity with long-term-care benefits. It is intended to solve or amelio-

5. It is also possible to purchase an increasing or variable immediate life annuity and a long-term-care insurance policy whose benefits increase at an annual rate of 5 percent. Purchase of policies with these features would address another risk factor—inflation—but, obviously, would be significantly more expensive.

rate many of the problems existing in the product markets as they are currently structured and operate. Moreover, because it solves a number of these product problems, it is claimed that, with the appropriate marketing and supporting governmental policies, an integrated insurance policy would, if widely purchased, substantially assist in the achievement of important public policy goals: reducing dependence on Medicaid and Medicare and enhancing the desirability of annuitization of a portion of household assets to protect against the risk of impoverishment in extreme old age.

The integrated product that my colleagues and I examined is a fixed immediate life annuity with payments that increase upon the determination of a severe disability. More specifically, we modeled a life annuity issued to a 65-year-old (gender-neutral) individual that pays $1,000 a month for life with a guaranteed ten-year minimum payout. It is integrated with a disability rider that pays an additional $2,000 a month if the insured becomes chronically disabled in at least two of six ADLs or is cognitively impaired for at least ninety days and an another additional $2,000 a month if the insured becomes disabled in four ADLs. These benefit levels are similar to the levels of the combination of products described above.

A single premium was estimated for this integrated product based on data from the 1986 National Mortality Follow-Back Study, which reports the disability and mortality experience of a sample of individuals from the general population. Small expense loadings were added to cover administrative costs, but almost no marketing expenses; the assumed discount rate is 6 percent, used in calculating the present expected value of benefits from age at the time of purchase to death. No lapses are assumed, because the integrated product is purchased with a single premium. The empirical analysis divides the population into two groups: one group, under current long-term-care underwriting practice, could purchase long-term-care insurance; it is assumed that, because of their good health, these individuals also are good proxies for current life-annuity purchasers. For the integrated product, we assume that the only individuals excluded from purchase would be those who would immediately claim disability benefits. We call this minimal underwriting; everyone else is deemed qualified to purchase the integrated product.

The empirical results shown in table 15-1 suggest that minimal underwriting dramatically increases the pool of eligible purchasers to 98 percent of persons at age 65, from 77 percent under current long-term-care insurance underwriting practice. The expansion has relatively modest impacts on mean risk and expected duration of disability in the prospective purchaser pool under minimal underwriting but reduces average survival by 1.5 years. Minimal underwriting excludes persons whose expected survival is only another six

Table 15-1. *Descriptive Statistics for Hypothetical Purchasers and Nonpurchasers of Immediate Life Annuity and Disability Benefits at Age 65*
Units as indicated

Category	Percent in risk category	Mean survival (years)	Percent meeting 2+ ADL benefit trigger	Expected years of 2+ ADL disability	Percent meeting 4+ ADL benefit trigger	Expected years of 4+ ADL disability
All persons	100.0	17.8	68.5	1.5	50.7	0.7
Purchasers						
Current annuitant proxies	77.1	19.5	69.0	1.5	51.6	0.7
Expanded purchase pool	98.0	18.0	67.9	1.4	50.2	0.6
Nonpurchasers						
Current long-term care underwriting practice	22.9	11.7	66.8	1.5	47.7	0.6
Minimal underwriting only	2.0	5.9	100.0	5.8	74.2	2.0

Source: Author's calculations based on data from Murtaugh, Spillman, and Warshawsky (2001).

Table 15-2. *Life Care Annuity Premium at Age 65, by Benefit Level and
Underwriting Practice*
Dollars

Recipient	$1,000 monthly life annuity only	$2,000 monthly 2+ ADL disability benefit	$2,000 monthly 4+ ADL disability benefit	Integrated premium
All persons	139,098	15,950	6,310	161,358
Prospective purchasers				
Current long-term care underwriting	145,041	13,900	5,686	164,627
Minimal underwriting only	139,827	13,723	5,554	159,104
Nonpurchasers				
Current long-term care underwriting	119,051	22,866	8,414	150,331
Minimal underwriting only	104,147	122,764	42,586	269,497

Source: Author's calculations based on data from Murtaugh, Spillman, and Warshawsky
(2001).

years, on average, but whose expected duration of disability is about four times
that of prospective purchasers.

Table 15-2 shows the single premiums for the three levels of benefit and a
combined single premium resulting from the likely purchases by the relevant
populations. The premium for the life annuity only, at $139,827, for the
expanded purchaser pool under minimal underwriting is 3.6 percent lower than
that for likely annuity purchasers because of the expanded pool's lower
average survival. (As explained above, we assume likely annuity purchasers
currently have the same life expectancy as those who would pass through
current long-term-care underwriting.) The premium for the disability benefits
is similar for the two purchase groups because minimal underwriting excludes
the persons representing the worst disability cost risks, and the remaining "poor
risks" currently unable to purchase long-term-care insurance actually have
slightly lower disability costs than those currently able to purchase the insurance.
Combined with the lower annuity costs of prospective purchasers under minimal
underwriting, the premium for the combined product is $159,104, almost 4
percent lower than the premiums we estimate for a life annuity and long-term-
care insurance, under current underwriting practice, sold separately.[6]

6. It can also be shown that an integrated product with the right balance of straight life
annuity, guaranteed period, and long-term-care benefits would be attractive enough to a
sufficient number of those currently excluded from purchasing long-term-care insurance
to achieve the results described here.

Table 15-3.   *Projected Impact of ADL Inflation on Premium Cost at Age 65,*
by Benefit Level
Ratio to base premium

Recipient	2+ ADL disability benefit	4+ ADL disability benefit	Integrated premium, immediate annuity plus disability benefits
	ADL inflation[a]		
All persons	1.47	1.46	1.06
Prospective purchasers			
Current annuitant proxies	1.40	1.40	1.04
Expanded purchase pool	1.56	1.41	1.06
Nonpurchasers			
Current long-term care			
underwriting	1.62	1.59	1.11
Minimal underwriting only	1.00	1.73	1.06
	Earlier benefits[b]		
All persons	1.09	1.15	1.01
Prospective purchasers			
Current annuitant proxies	1.10	1.15	1.01
Expanded purchase pool	1.11	1.16	1.01
Nonpurchasers			
Current long-term care			
underwriting	1.07	1.13	1.01
Minimal underwriting only	1.00	1.04	1.00

Source: Author's calculations based on data from Murtaugh, Spillman, and Warshawsky (2001).

a. Assumes that all those with one ADL disability would obtain certification for two and those with three ADL disabilities would obtain certification for four if disability benefits were available.

b. Assumes that certification for chronic two-ADL and four-ADL disability would be obtained three months earlier if disability benefits were available.

The top panel of table 15-3 shows the percentage increases in premium in the event of what we call "ADL inflation," whereby individuals with one ADL impairment claim two ADLs and those with three such impairments claim four. This inflation, or "creep," represents two realistic considerations: the data in the National Mortality Follow-Back Study may somewhat underreport disabilities, and, more significantly, the existence of insurance coverage itself will tend to cause an increase in disability claims (so-called moral hazard). Including these considerations in the estimate increases the cost of the long-term-care benefits and raises the single premium for the integrated product to $169,066. This happens to be less than the $171,511 cost for a "do-it-yourself" combination available in the market. Because of the reduction in adverse selection, we also estimate it to be less than the combined cost of the two stand-alone products.

According to Mark Pauly, pure economic theory says that, in the absence of a Medicaid program, many households would have a preference for a life annuity with extra benefits payable following the onset of disability.[7] On practical marketing grounds, the integration of the two components, a life annuity and long-term-care insurance, is mutually reinforcing: the life annuity is no longer viewed as illiquid, and the long-term-care insurance no longer needs to be purchased at a young age to avoid potential underwriting problems. Moreover, integration reduces adverse selection in the life annuity and the need for extensive underwriting in long-term-care insurance: the integrated product is available at a lower cost to more people. The premium is guaranteed by the issuer and is not subject to post hoc increases. The disability benefit is more flexible. Finally, from the issuing insurance company's point of view, there is probably a reduction in actuarial risk coming from integration, as unexpectedly positive trends in life expectancy would be accompanied by a reduction in disability rates in most likely scenarios.

The Public Policy Environment

It is difficult to know exactly what the current policy environment is toward a product that does not yet exist. Yet certain problems and issues can be anticipated as inferred from first principles and from recent experience with related product innovations.

Taxation

A critical public policy issue is the taxation of the integrated product. For this purpose, one possible view would break the product, despite its essentially integrated nature, into its component parts—the life annuity and long-term-care insurance. If sold as tandem insurance contracts, which can be bought separately but are cheaper when bought together (as claimed above), then each would be taxed separately. If the product is purchased using after-tax money, payments from the life-annuity component presumably would be taxed using the current regime of the exclusion ratio.

The long-term-care insurance component is more difficult to evaluate. If the insurance policy were thought to be a single-premium product, as modeled in this example, then its premium would not be deductible because it would

7. Pauly (1990).

exceed the age-dependent limits. If the policy were thought to be paid through a flow of premiums (at a guaranteed level), then if it were deemed to be qualified, its premiums could be deductible, although subject, under current law, to a requirement that total medical expenses (including these insurance premiums) exceed 7.5 percent of adjusted gross income. In any case, payments from the qualified long-term-care component of the policy would not be taxable.

An alternative tax viewpoint would not break the integrated product into component parts. Rather, as primarily a life annuity, it would be taxed entirely as an annuity. If it were purchased with after-tax money, a pro rata portion of cost would be excluded from taxable income over life expectancy. Any proceeds from the long-term-care insurance component would be taxable. If the integrated product were purchased using pretax money from a qualified retirement plan, then the life-annuity payments would be subject to income taxation. The premium (or premiums) for the long-term-care insurance component would presumably be considered a nontaxable investment, but the distribution of the insurance policy would be included in taxable income. If the policy were not distributed, then all payments would be taxed; but in that case section 401(a)(9)—minimum distribution rule—issues would arise, and this too is an area currently in flux and uncertain in these regards. Qualified long-term-care expenses are deductible to the extent that medical expenses exceed 7.5 percent of adjusted gross income.

An alternative tax approach might view the integrated product within a retirement plan as analogous to a 401(h) plan, which provides retirement income as well as health benefits to plan participants. As above, life-annuity payments would be taxable. The "purchase" of the long-term-care insurance would not be considered a taxable distribution. Long-term-care benefits paid from the policy would not be included in taxable income. Clearly, this latter approach is more tax favored.[8]

Medicaid

Partnership programs are currently allowed and functioning in four states. Under these programs, which have achieved a modest degree of penetration in the elderly population, if the benefits under an individual's "qualified" long-term-care insurance policy were to run out, he or she could be eligible for

---

8. Proposals to tax the payments from a life annuity, whether nonqualified or qualified, at capital gains rates have also been made; such tax treatment would presumably apply to all the components of a life care annuity.

Medicaid in that state without incurring the strictures of spend-down rules. There are proposals to extend these programs across the nation. The long-term-care insurance policy qualifying for the program is required to provide benefits lasting only two or three years. Obviously, such a policy is cheaper than a lifetime benefit policy, and therefore it is presumably cheaper than the long-term-care insurance component of the integrated product under discussion here. Therefore, partnership programs, as currently constituted, would discourage the sales of the integrated product. One possible solution to this nascent problem would be to allow life care annuities with short-duration long-term-care benefit features to be eligible for partnership programs. Another solution would be to have Medicaid pick up the long-term-care expenses that are not covered by an integrated product. For example, in the product illustrated above (which did not increase benefits with inflation), a partnership would have the insurance policy pay out its benefits but then have Medicaid pay for the extra costs of care incurred owing to inflation in the cost of long-term-care services since the time the policy was issued.

Insurance Laws

The life annuity is regulated by state insurance commissions as a life insurance product. Long-term-care insurance is regulated by state insurance commissions as a health insurance product. The policy concerns relating to these two product groups are different in many dimensions, and therefore the regulatory stances toward them are different, as well. When a product combines features from these two worlds, the insurance regulator is faced with some perplexing issues and must take some time to grapple with them. This apparently has been the experience of some new integrated insurance products. It clearly represents a barrier to introducing the life care annuity unless some regulatory understandings are achieved before introduction of the product.

Administrative Issues

We have modeled and advocated a disability approach to the long-term-care insurance component of the life care annuity. Although there are certain clear advantages to disability-dependent cash benefits, there are also certain disadvantages, which is why few insurance companies take such an approach in the design of their insurance policies. In particular, moral hazard, or the tendency of the insureds to exaggerate their rights to claim benefits under an insurance policy, is more likely to be a problem in a disability policy than in an indemnity or expense reimbursement policy, under which, for example, an individual must enter a nursing home, as well as be disabled, to get benefits. It should be noted, however, that a cash disability approach does not cause an increase in the utilization of particular services, as an expense reimbursement policy might.

The likely response of the insurance company to the moral hazard problem is either to accept its existence or to institute strict claims review and monitoring practices; either way leads to higher premium rates. A possible solution to this issue in the context of the life care annuity would be to allow the long-term-care insurance component to utilize, perhaps at the option of the insured, indemnity or expense reimbursement approaches. Another possible solution is in product design that would discourage early claiming—for example, a schedule in the policy whereby the level of disability benefits payable increases with age.

Conclusion

Although, for most households, the private sector is the appropriate primary place to address issues surrounding long-term-care financing and retirement income security, actual products sold in the market have some drawbacks. That is why I have proposed the life care annuity, an integrated insurance product, which empirical research summarized here has shown to be a better approach in cost and availability dimensions. Yet some challenges, especially in the tax area, and unresolved narrower policy issues might pose difficulties to the actual introduction of the product. I also believe, however, that the time for action has arrived, that these challenges should be met, and that the ideas proposed in this paper should be tested in the market through actual introduction of the life care annuity. I have discussed the product mainly in terms of an individually marketed product because that is where most innovations occur, where new ideas can be more easily tested, and it is, besides, the focus of current market attention. Yet it is also possible to envision this idea's application to group annuities in pension plans and to individual accounts in a reformed Social Security system. One demonstration possibility would be to introduce the life care annuity as an option for federal employee retirement plans.

At the same time as action is taken, further analysis is appropriate and indeed has begun. Murtaugh, Spillman, and I are currently using the 1993 National Mortality Follow-Back Study to update and expand our empirical analysis. A large project being undertaken at Georgetown University, sponsored by the Robert Wood Johnson Foundation, is examining the public policy aspects of long-term care by exploring several different policy proposals, including the life care annuity. As part of those examinations, the populations that, by socioeconomic characteristics, are most likely to benefit from and utilize the integrated product will be studied. I believe that these are all fruitful avenues of exploration that should proceed at the same time as we gain more practical information from the actual introduction of a new insurance product into the marketplace, one that meets the real needs of a growing segment of our population.

References

Brown, Jeffrey, and others. 2001. *The Role of Annuity Markets in Financing Retirement*. MIT Press.

Murtaugh, Christopher, Brenda Spillman, and Mark Warshawsky. 2001. "In Sickness and in Health: An Annuity Approach to Financing Long-Term Care and Retirement Income." *Journal of Risk and Insurance* 68 (2): 225–54.

Pauly, Mark V. 1990. "The Rational Nonpurchase of Long-Term-Care Insurance." *Journal of Political Economy* 98 (1): 153–68.

16

Long-Term Care for the Elderly: Lessons from Abroad

Mark Merlis

A COMPARISON OF long-term-care systems from selected countries can yield useful models of reform for the United States. It is important to observe from the start, however, that most countries do not have coherent long-term-care systems that we could somehow imitate or import. What happens to the dependent elderly in each country is the outcome of a complex of historic choices in health policy, pension policy, and housing policy. It is, therefore, less useful to talk about whole systems than about specific features of those systems (table 16-1).

A few overly broad generalizations may be helpful to begin a comparison. Most countries still have, as we do, what can be labeled a social assistance model: in each case, public assistance for long-term care started out as a subset of assistance for the indigent elderly and has continued to reflect that historic welfare basis. It is really only in the past ten years that a few countries—most prominently, Germany and Japan—have moved in the direction of social insurance, a population-wide entitlement that some people call a third pillar of protection, alongside pensions and health care. Of course, there have been all along a handful of cradle-to-grave welfare states, which have much more extensive public provision, though they are facing increasing constraints and downsizing—to the point that a private long-term-care insurance market has emerged in Sweden. On the other hand, some countries—Spain and Italy, for example, and, until recently, Austria—still have only a tiny formal long-term-care sector and a much stronger expectation that extended families will take care of their own elderly.

I touch on the German and Japanese systems only briefly, partly because they have had much attention in other forums and partly because the United States is unlikely to adopt their long-term-care systems any time soon. Both the German and Japanese systems are funded through what are called premiums but amount to fixed-rate payroll and pension taxes. These apply to virtually

Table 16-1. *Basic Features of Long-Term-Care Financing Models, Selected OECD Countries*

Model	Countries	Means tested	Funding	Benefits
Social assistance	United States and most other OECD countries	Yes	General revenue	Service
Social insurance	Germany, Japan	No	Earmarked revenue	Budget for services
Classic welfare state	Norway, Sweden	No	General revenue	Service
Family provision, minimal public contribution	Spain, Italy	. . .	. . .	. . .

everyone in Germany, in Japan only to people age 40 and over, and they are supplemented with general funds from both central and local governments. Even with earmarked funding sources, the systems are basically pay-as-you-go. Germany may be building a little surplus for the time being, but there is no expectation that current workers are somehow saving for their future needs. Both systems have disability thresholds for benefits, and both assign people to classes, based on ascending levels of disability, and give each class a fixed budget to spend on services, not an open-ended entitlement. In Germany, noninstitutionalized people can opt to take a lesser amount as cash, and most people have done so.

A couple of other countries—Austria and the Netherlands—have gone part of the way toward social insurance, and a whole lot more have been flirting with the idea for years but have not implemented such a plan, for various reasons. A commission in the United Kingdom proposed sweeping reforms in 1998, but the subject has taken a back seat to the more urgent political issue of reforming the National Health Service. The federal government in Canada floated a proposal under which increased funding to provincial systems would have been accompanied by some uniform protections for home care, which is not part of the basic Medicare guarantee; the provinces wanted money without any such strings. Protracted debate in other countries has focused on issues that are familiar in the United States: public versus personal responsibility, national and local roles, in-cash versus in-kind benefits.

In sum, most countries are still on the social assistance model, and their systems broadly resemble ours in the following respects:

Table 16-2.   *Public Share of Long-Term-Care Spending, Selected OECD Countries, 1992–95*

Percent

Country	Share of spending
United States	53
Belgium	55
Netherlands	67
Canada	70
United Kingdom	77
Finland	79
Australia	81
Norway	100
Sweden	100

Source: Author's calculations based on data from Jacobzone (1998).

—universal medical coverage that includes only limited long-term-care benefits,

—a parallel and distinct long-term-care system that tends to be operated by local governments with varying degrees of central government funding,

—at least some degree of means testing, and

—some amount of rationing, or underprovision, or at least a perception of unmet need.

The following discussion focuses on a few key issues: the mix of public and private money, how services are rationed, housing, and informal caregiving.

Table 16-2 gives estimates of the public sector share of spending on long-term care in various countries—basically a spectrum, with the United States at one end, Sweden at the other, and seven other countries in between. Unfortunately, these percentages are old, many countries' data are unreported, and the comparisons are fraught with definitional problems. For example, in the United States, individuals who sign over their Social Security checks to a nursing home are classified as making self-payments, thus placing them in the private category. In some other countries, when the government begins paying for a person's nursing-home care, it no longer sends the patient a pension check. These two circumstances really amount to the same thing. If the data in table 16-2 were corrected for that, the United States would probably be a little closer to the middle. Other systems differ from ours not just in the relative private share but, more important, in the forms those private contributions take.

The United States has what could be described as a before-and-after system of cost sharing: Those in need of long-term care pay for everything—in effect, 100 percent co-payment—until they have exhausted their resources. Then, after they have impoverished themselves, the government steps in. The alternative to this kind of brutal chronological system is one in which, from the outset, the government and the individual both pay a share. For example, some systems have a sliding income-based scale for coinsurance; this is true in Belgium and the Netherlands. Alternatively, a system can have level coinsurance rates but an income-based annual cap on coinsurance. In Finland, for example, there is a protected income level below which the individual pays nothing; if an individual's income is above that level, he or she pays out-of-pocket no more than 35 percent of the excess income. In effect, it is a sort of partial spend-down. Some countries have moved away from asset tests. For example, the Netherlands used to have an asset spend-down requirement for institutional care; now it has only income-based charges. France has no asset testing, but it does have estate recovery.

Finally, there is at least some trend toward thinking of care—both skilled and unskilled—as a service that ought to receive the same level of public support regardless of whether the recipient is at home or in some kind of institution. Under this thinking, the individual remains responsible for room and board, and maybe cleaning, regardless of setting. In short, there may be more rational and less draconian ways of extracting money from patients that could be adopted in the United States without dramatically changing the overall mix.

Rationing exists to some degree everywhere; not everybody is getting every service needed or nominally covered. Some of this rationing is formal: disability thresholds for services, deliberate limitation of bed supply or home-care slots. In at least a couple of countries, however, local agencies operating under budget constraints decide who gets what on a more informal basis, looking not just at the level of disability but also at where an individual lives, what kind of social supports he or she has, and so on. The United States is much too legalistic for anything as arbitrary as that, but if we are going to ration we might at least try to think about assessment systems that could prioritize on the basis of the totality of an individual's circumstances instead of just counting the number of activities of daily living with which the individual requires assistance.

Table 16-3 compares housing places for the elderly in a few countries for which data are available. Some housing categories used elsewhere are not typically applied in the United States, and some of the figures for the United States are rough equivalents. The table suggests that the combined number of institutional and social housing units does not vary much between countries, but the United States has been much more reliant on the most intensive setting—nursing homes—than the other countries. Other countries are more likely to have public funding for places called old-age homes or hostels, and they tend to have a bigger investment in various kinds of public or subsidized

Table 16-3. *Institutional and Social Publicly Funded Housing for People Aged 65 or Older in Selected OECD Countries, Various Years*
Units per 100 persons

Country	Nursing home	Old-age home	Social housing	Total
Sweden (1995)	1.8	2.9	4.0	8.7
France (1996)	1.6	4.5	1.8	7.9
United Kingdom (1994)	1.8	3.1	5.0	9.9
Netherlands (1994)	2.6	6.4	2.3	11.3
United States (1998)[a]	5.3	2.6	1.2	9.1

Source: Pacolet and others (2000) for European data; author's calculations of data from Harrington and others (2000) and U.S. Department of Housing and Urban Developing, "Housing Our Elders" (www.huduser.org/publications/hsgspec/housec.html [September 2002] for U.S. data).

a. For the United States, "old-age home" is defined as any state-licensed residential facility other than a nursing home, excluding facilities for the nonaged (for example, those for the mentally retarded or mentally ill, for substance abuse, or for persons with AIDS). "Social housing" is defined as a public housing unit occupied by a household headed by a person aged 62 or older.

housing for the elderly that provides at least some social services. I do not know if there is a lesson here, except that there may be some irreducible proportion of people who cannot stay in their own homes, and we may need to explore ways of shifting more public resources toward intermediate alternatives. Further research is needed on this question and to obtain data from additional countries.

Finally, a number of countries have concerns similar to ours about maintaining informal caregiving. A few countries directly pay family members for services or count the time they spend on caregiving toward retirement, which is important under some systems. In others, money goes directly to the elderly person, and he or she can use it to compensate family members. In these programs, either the number of participants is limited or the amounts involved are too small to adequately compensate those who have to reduce their labor-force participation, so it is not clear that they have had much impact. Giving greater emphasis to nonfinancial support for caregiving, such as the extensive respite care provided in Germany and Australia, may prove a productive innovation. Australia's caregiver package includes education and counseling and various other supports. Finally, a number of countries still provide what amount to negative incentives for family caregiving. They require family members to make financial contributions to care. Austria, for example can obligate people to pay for their siblings' care. Other countries may explicitly limit formal home care when a spouse or other relative is living in the home.

Whether these policies actually increase the amount of family caregiving is not clear.

To sum up, since the United States is unlikely to enact social insurance in the near future, there are a few areas in which it might be useful to look at policies in Europe and elsewhere as models for incremental measures. These models may help us come up with more reasonable systems of income-based patient cost sharing, for example. Furthermore, we can look for ways of rationing or prioritizing that are more sensitive to people's overall needs and circumstances. Additionally, we can start exploring housing policy as a key component of planning for caring for the elderly. Finally, we can do more to support informal caregiving.

References

Harrington, Charlene, and others. 2000. *1998 State Data Book on Long-Term Care Program and Market Characteristics.* San Francisco: University of California, Department of Social and Behavioral Sciences.

Jacobzone, Stephane, and others. 1998. *Long-Term Care Services to Older People, a Perspective on Future Needs: The Impact of An* [sic] *Improving Health of Older Persons.* Ageing Working Paper AWP 4.2. Paris: Organization for Economic Cooperation and Development.

Pacolet, Jozef, and others. 2000. *Social Protection for Dependency in Old Age: A Study of the Fifteen EU Member States and Norway.* Aldershot, England: Ashgate.

17

Caring Communities:
What Would It Take?

Deborah Stone

WHEN WE ARE OLD, or when we are in need of help, we hope for loving care. When we need help caring for our parents, our children, or our sisters and brothers, we hope that the people who help us care for them are loving, too. Against all these hopes, we are tormented by a recurring nightmare: that we will end our days in a nursing home, or that someday we will have to put someone we love into one.

Care begins at home, in the family, among people who love one another. That kind of care is the most private and intimate and the kind we most cherish. At the other end is public care, the stuff we know by ugly names like long-term care, home- and community-based services, and skilled-nursing facilities, with its unfortunately pungent acronym, SNF. Simple words like *love* and *care* are notably absent from the public vocabulary. This discrepancy in the very language of care is only the surface crack of a deep chasm between the public and private worlds of caring, between our hopes and our nightmares.

Reality, of course, is far more complex than hopes and nightmares. It always is. Family caregiving begins in love and loyalty and springs from the heart before the head, but it can quickly become burdensome, conflictual, even hellish. Caregiving can drive people apart, strain marriages, fracture families. At the other end of the spectrum, public care, the care given by strangers trained in technique and beholden to accountants, can start out cold and distant but quickly ripen into loving, almost familial relationships.

Yet on the whole, there is a long distance between the kind of care we wish for ourselves and our families and the kind of care we are willing and able to provide for our fellow citizens. That the public sector sometimes has to help us in our private lives is a given. The questions we face are how and whether it is possible to make care in the public sector live up to our private ideals. Can we envision a world in which getting care for ourselves or someone we love is not a nightmare? Is there some place between the ideal world of family care (which is often anything but idyllic) and the public world of institutional and program-matic care (which certainly has its glorious moments)? Is it possible to envision a caring community that can support family caregivers without displacing them altogether but without exploiting them, either?

"Caring community" is my shorthand for a space that offers the security of public responsibility and protection but also the warmth and intimacy that we imagine, and often practice, in families. Government and policymakers usually approach these issues by resolving to make changes in the way care is paid for, the way personnel are trained, the way quality is regulated and monitored. Caring communities cannot be created, however, simply by rounding up the usual suspects—pay, personnel, and procedures. Those of us in the policy arena need to change our thinking by stepping outside ourselves as policymakers and analysts and adopting instead the insider perspective—or, rather, three insider perspectives: first, the person who needs and gets care; second, family caregivers, who are the first line of defense and sometimes the constant presence; and third, direct-care workers, the aides at the bottom of the totem pole in the formal system, those who actually do the hands-on care.

Caring communities would embody the values of these people instead of the values of economists, managers, and planners. From the insider perspective, the most basic policy assumptions anchoring our system of long-term care appear warped.

Policy Assumption 1: Care Can Be Rationalized and Made More Efficient

A home-care aide told me she was once reprimanded by her supervisor for taking too long with an elderly client. All the client really needed, it seems, was help putting on her elastic stockings. The aide billed thirty minutes for the visit. Her supervisor thought she ought to have been able to do it in ten. The aide saw the episode as emblematic of the trouble with home health care: "You can't just go in and get out. I'm sorry. You know, my grandmother had people taking care of her. I wouldn't want them to do the same—you know, just come in and wash her up and leave. They have to have some kind of relationship going."[1]

A policy analyst or manager might well agree with the supervisor. From that perspective, the aide's leisurely approach is just the sort of featherbedding public and private payers should be snuffing out. I would suggest, however,

1. Unless otherwise noted, anecdotes from interviews are from research I did in 1998–2000 and more fully reported in Stone (2000a and 2000b).

that the incident is emblematic of something else. It hints at the industrial revolution in care. Caregiving, like textile weaving, used to be done in private homes, mostly by women, using simple methods handed down through generations and learned at the hearth. Women gave care as it was needed, as they thought best, as they were moved by their sense of obligation and their concern for the people around them.[2]

Over the course of the twentieth century, a lot of caregiving moved out of the home into hospitals and institutions that were often called homes (nursing homes, Homes for Little Wanderers, group homes) but were in fact more like factories. At the same time, a lot of caring work (though not all—most is still done by families)[3] was organized into formal occupations with training and licensing requirements and with somebody higher up calling the shots—prescribing care plans, dictating schedules and pay scales, and generally controlling the content of care. Care became a service and, like most services, was now another kind of economic commodity, to be produced and packaged, bought and sold, counted and hoarded.

In the early twentieth century, Frederick Winslow Taylor went into the factory, timed the workers at their tasks, watched them carefully, and broke down their work into minute gestures and steps. He figured out the quickest, most efficient way for workers do their jobs and then reconstituted those jobs, training workers with a stopwatch and standardizing the human components of work as much as possible, eliminating all quirks, spontaneity, and, most of all, independent thinking and judgment.

Prospective payment for home-care agencies and nursing homes takes Taylorization one step further. In the Taylor-inspired factory, a functional task was broken down into discrete physical motions. Now, in long-term care, people are reduced to their illnesses or disabilities, chalked off on a home-care admissions chart or squeezed into discrete nursing diagnostic categories. Their illnesses are then broken down into care tasks. Somewhere in computer land, someone models which tasks need to be done for the average person in each category; in professional argot, a patient classification system predicts resource utilization. Somewhere (is it Washington?), someone figures out how much money all this care (now called resource utilization) ought to cost—or at any rate, how much government is willing to pay for it. Before you know it, a woman is only a body that needs elastic stockings.

The stocking story is chilling because it captures the transformation of care into a package of standardized tasks and the transformation of the patient into

2. A wonderful history of family caregiving is *Hearts of Wisdom* (Abel 2001).
3. Arno, Levine, and Memmott (2000).

an object to which tasks are done.[4] Officially, the home health visit no longer represents a relationship, or even part of a relationship, between the giver and the recipient of care. The visit has become a container for discrete tasks—physical, observable, documentable, measurable tasks. When home health aides make a visit, especially if they are employed by agencies and even more especially if the client's care is paid for by third parties, they go into the home with a checklist, a plan, that tells them exactly what tasks they are supposed to do—no more, no less. When aides make the rounds in a nursing home, they, too, work by the book. Someone else has already decided what should be done for each patient and, often, how much time should be allotted for each task. Even if no one has actually decided or prescribed how much time it takes to put on elastic hose or give a person his pills, the workload assigned to aides is a de facto allocation of their time.

Standardization is the way of modern management. Quality and efficiency, policy analysts are taught, are gained by discerning common patterns and using simplifying rules. Moreover, this way of controlling costs is believed to have the supreme virtue of allowing caregivers discretion. They can provide whatever care they think necessary, including building relationships—as long as they stay within the budget. The only trouble is, in most cases, the reimbursement amounts do not begin to cover even half of what caregivers think their patients need.

The stocking story suggests one way policymakers ought to change in how they think about long-term-care policy. Care involves more than procedures. It involves relationships as well as tasks. For most people, in fact, the quality of the relationship is the most important element of care. Most people experience their need for help as an assault on their dignity. The extra twenty minutes an aide spends talking to a woman before helping her with a bodily task can sustain her identity as a person with a life and a history, loves and hurts, accomplishments and failures, hopes and fears—something other than a body that needs fixing up, emptying, cleaning, and feeding.

Policy Assumption 2: Better Data Are the Key to Improving Care

There is a truism in long-term care that first visits are more costly than later visits. Whether it is hospice care, a nursing home, or home care, everybody

---

4. Actually, the stocking story is from the days just before prospective payment went into effect, so it illustrates how much the mentality of Taylor's scientific management had already permeated home care, even before the Taylorites enacted their reforms.

agrees the intake visit takes longer and costs more—as well it should. From the perspective of care recipients, though, the values are reversed. The thirtieth visit is often much more valuable than the first because, by then, a relationship has been built, and the caregiver is able to make the client feel like more than merely a case. Even before the new prospective payment system went into effect in home care, requiring a long survey on the first visit, the initial home-care visit was typically a two-hour affair. Although it was costly to an agency, it was nearly useless to clients, who simply answered questions and signed lots of forms giving their consent to things over which they had no control anyway, such as allowing information to go to an insurer and agreeing not to sue anybody.

My mother once had home care from a visiting nurse after some major surgery. I had brought her home from the hospital and was there when the nurse came. I valiantly fought all my urges to do field research on my mother and gave her privacy with the nurse. Two hours later, as soon as the nurse was out the door, I couldn't wait to ask Mom what the visit was like. "She didn't do a damn thing," my mother grumbled. "All she did was ask questions and take notes."

As a researcher who has studied home health care, I *know* what the nurse did that day. She gathered data, lots of it, for better patient assessment, better risk adjustment (another code word for predicting resource utilization), and better ability to measure outcomes and quality down the line. She would also use all that data to better "integrate" and "coordinate" my mother's care. She "informed" my mother about her choices and got her "informed consent" to treatment. My mother, on pain medication and still in a postanesthesia stupor, was hardly in a position to make informed decisions about anything. No matter. The visiting nurse gave my mother the toll-free hotline number to report any suspected fraud to the Office of the Inspector General. The nurse also created an electronic record by typing all the information directly into a laptop computer, the better to integrate my mother's care.

The visiting nurse was doing all the things that policy analysts agree are necessary to improve the quality of long-term care. Yet on the day my mother came home from the hospital, the day she was most frightened and most in need of reassurance and explanations and a little human warmth, her first and longest contact with home health care amounted to "not a damn thing." The nurse massaged her laptop and never once touched Mom.

Policy Assumption 3: Managers and Analysts Are the Most Valuable Players in Long-Term Care

A few years ago, I met with the chair of my university's political science department to discuss my future research plans. The man studies presidents, political parties, and elections—the usual topics of political science. I worried that when I told him I was studying home health care, he would think I had gone mushy and was a lost cause to his stellar department. Instead, he told me a story: His mother had had a home health aide for a long time before she died, and at his mother's funeral, he insisted that the aide ride in the limousine with the family. "She was my mother's best friend, the most important person to her, and I wanted her to have a place of honor."

In our long-term-care systems, no one is asking the lowly aides to ride in the limo. But the fact is, the person who is the least qualified and skilled member of the staff from the chief executive's perspective is often the most skilled, qualified, and valuable to the patient and, for that matter, to the patient's family. Yet frontline care workers are the lowest paid in the industry. The more training and degrees workers have, the less contact they have with patients and clients; the less contact they have with patients and clients, the more they are paid and the better they are rewarded.

In the industrial model, this hierarchy makes a certain sense (though even there, it comes under challenge): the most skilled and valuable work is performed by the people at the top—the brains: the managers, executives, planners, and professionals. These are the people Robert Reich calls "symbolic analysts." They manipulate symbols and abstractions. They see through particulars and individuality and uniqueness to the generalizable essence of things.[5] Unfortunately, in caregiving, symbolic analysts see right through the people who need care—and you cannot take good care of somebody you do not see.

What matters most to care recipients is how they are treated by frontline workers, the people who are at the bottom in the industrial model. Social workers or case managers may think they know how long it takes an aide to dress a client or to give a bath; a computer model may even think it knows how long it takes to dress and bathe five patients. Neither the case manager nor the computer, however, knows what the aide knows: exactly how a client's body moves and tires, where it aches, how to modify a standard routine to fit each client's needs. Nurses and doctors may have standards to guide them in setting up a care plan or may take such standards from carefully worked-out packages prepared by professional care planners. But it is the aide who knows the subtle arts of coaxing, joking, and soothing people into complying with the pieces of the plan.

Of course, policy matters. Eligibility for services is a matter of great moment to home-care clients. Whether Medicare will pay for Grandma's

5. Reich (1998).

nursing-home care is a decision of cataclysmic importance to her family. However, as Michael Lipsky pointed out long ago, from the perspective of the ordinary citizen gingerly entering a bureaucracy in need of help, the greatest power sits not in the corporate suite on the hundredth floor but down at street level, where gatekeepers decide the fates of supplicants, one by one.[6]

It is another truism that aides and nursing assistants are underpaid, woefully underpaid. Many policy analysts are thinking about how to upgrade these workers' pay and how to build career ladders and other devices to stem their extraordinarily high turnover rates. Little progress will be made on this front until policymakers and analysts get inside the perspective of care recipients and families and reenvision the work of care. Only from this perspective is it obvious that the people at the bottom of traditional hierarchies of skill, training, and authority are in fact at the top in terms of the care they give.

In a caring community, aides would ride in the limo. They would be paid something closer to what they are worth, and they would be made part of team meetings and case planning conferences. They would be taught not only how to protect their backs but also how to make their voices heard, how to articulate their patients' problems and needs.

Policy Assumption 4: Overutilization of Care Is a Big Problem

Much of the literature on Medicare and long-term care suggests that the biggest problem is excessive use: costs have skyrocketed because utilization has zoomed, and utilization has zoomed because too many patients are too quick to run for help and too many providers see a chance to make money by helping them. Most of the policy developments in the past fifteen years are aimed at curbing use of services. One would have to ferret deep into the collective memory bank to learn that the same government that now discourages use of long-term care services once touted first nursing homes and then home health care as cheaper alternatives to hospital care.

But memory fades as the polity ages, and now the reigning collective wisdom holds that because users do not have to pay for home health care themselves, they have no reason to hold down its use.[7] Co-payment, it is said, is necessary to encourage patients and families to evaluate the worth of care with a more realistic eye. In policy jargon, this is referred to as "setting the

6. Lipsky (1988).
7. This is almost dogma, repeated with the monotonous regularity of catechism among government officials and policy analysts alike; see Stone (2000, p. 18).

proper incentives," but what is really meant is discouraging people from availing themselves of help.

This theory makes sense only if we view long-term care as a good in the economic sense. In the economic sense, a good is a commodity or service that benefits people and enhances their welfare. According to the law of demand, people will consume more of a good if they can get it for less—or better yet, for nothing. Care, however, is not an unalloyed good. Home-care services do have value to people, sometimes very precious value but they are never unequivocally good. Few people want to be in a position to need home care, or medical care of any kind, and even fewer consider residence in a nursing-home as a good they are eager to consume. To seek help is to cast oneself as dependent, but American culture reveres independence, and in such a culture dependence is humiliating. Shame, humiliation, and the loss of one's autonomy are the ever-present deterrents to using care. Money isn't the half of it.

Home health aides have consistently told me that new clients hate to have help showering or bathing and frequently refuse to let an aide bathe them for weeks. I asked one aide if this was more often problem with men than with women, since aides are mostly women. "Oh, no," she said. "Both. Every single person says 'I haven't been bathed this way since I was a child. It really hurts my pride. It hurts my dignity'."

Family caregivers caring for their elderly parents or declining spouses know all too well how hard it is to persuade someone to accept care even absent the money issue. One of my friends watched her husband struggle to pick up a book he had dropped on the floor, then silently cry in frustration. He had had a hip replacement, and though he had every reason to expect full recovery, he would sooner put himself in pain and exhaust himself doing a simple task than ask his wife for help and make himself dependent on her.

A caring community would not fear exploitation of its capacity to care. It would not regard people who need care as predators on the common weal. Instead of erecting fences to limit access to care, it would ensure that its members could seek the help they need without threat to their dignity. In a caring community, dependence and the care it requires would be natural features of life rather than a badge of shame.

Policy Assumption 5: Compassion Must Be Balanced with Hard-Nosed Fiscal Realism

The Balanced Budget Act of 1997 introduced prospective payment into Medicare home health care. A year later, without any sense of irony, the clinical director of a home-care agency told me that since its passage, her agency has had to "balance" short-term and long-term patients. She does not, for example, accept a patient leaving the hospital with chronic-care needs; she tells the hospital discharge planner that such placement would be "inappropriate." The owner of a Minnesota home-care agency was more blunt: "We will not take on a client who will be a six-month client because Medicare will not pay for it."[8]

Alongside the assumption that consumers are all too eager to consume long-term care, our long-term-care policy assumes that people in the business of caregiving are all too eager to *give* care. Prospective payment is nothing if not a system designed to curb caregivers' compassion. Prospective payment is a Ulysses contract: Ulysses had himself tied to the mast so he would be unable to respond to the siren calls that he knew he could not resist of his own free will.

Without a firm limit on reimbursement, policymakers believe, nurses, doctors, agencies, social workers, planners—anyone in a position to hear the siren calls of suffering—might be unable to control the impulse to help. Caregivers are famously incapable of closing the door on people in need. So prospective payment tells caregivers, "This much we will pay for. Any more you do out of your own pocket." Prospective payment is designed to make care providers husband their care, close their doors, and wheedle someone else— Medicaid, state waiver programs, or family members—into helping those in need.

Home-care nurses and administrators told me much about the increased importance of "planning" once prospective payment went into effect. "What kind of planning?" I would always ask. *Planning* turned out to be a euphemism for determining whether there were relatives who could take the patient in or whether the patient was eligible for Medicaid or the state waiver program. Planning, in short, means finding somebody *else* to take care of the patient.

Caregiving is a generous act. It is also addictive: people who start caring for others have a hard time stopping. Compassion feeds on itself. Whether family caregiving or paid caregiving, all the instincts are to give, to respond to the suffering of others. Very sick, frail, and disabled people have nearly unlimited needs. In the private realm, these needs can hijack a caregiver's life. In the public realm, they can hijack the public budget. Caregivers need ways to protect themselves in both the private and public realms.

For all the expansionary pressures of care needs, however, the rules are sometimes so rigid that they prevent people and institutions from responding to

8. Reported in Glenn Howatt, "Home Care Agencies Face a New Challenge," *Star Tribune* (Minneapolis), April 12, 1999, p. A1.

need. Caring communities have to strike a balance between permitting discretion and protecting caregivers from overwhelming demands. The supports that protect caregivers must be flexible enough to allow them to express compassion and to allow the community to expand its generosity.

Policy Assumption 6: Love Is Taboo

Emily Abel and Margaret Nelson, sisters who are both academic social scientists and who study caregiving, had to hire someone to take care of their widowed father as he became more disabled and sick. They hired Jasmine, a woman their mother had first taken on as a housekeeper. Gradually, they asked Jasmine to do more and more personal care of their father, ultimately bathing him and helping him go to the toilet. When the question arose where their father should spend his final weeks, the sisters suddenly understood that "Jasmine had become more important than any of his children and that he had to remain where she could see him every day. We could reminisce and try to enact old roles, but she related to him on the basis of the life they shared together."[9]

As I interviewed home-care workers, from nurses and therapists to aides, I was most struck by how much they used the word love when talking about their clients. Caring and being cared for often create an intimate relationship. People in these formal caregiving relationships often come to feel like kin. Indeed, it is not unusual these days to read an obituary and find a caregiver listed among those left behind by the deceased.

Love is not a word that rolls easily off the tongue in policy settings. In fact we are scared of it, terrified. We are terrified because, like the unbounded needs of patients that threaten to devour budgets, love suggests the unbounded compassion of caregivers that threatens to defy all management controls. Either one could bankrupt the national treasury if not nipped in the bud.

Moreover, love is—ahem—unprofessional. One abiding lesson of professional education is the supreme importance of keeping one's distance. The good professional caregiver does not have favorites and does not get too attached (though it is never made clear just how attached is too attached). In my research, nurses, therapists, and aides reported that during their training, they were told not to share personal information with clients. They were warned against getting too close and against becoming emotionally involved. Nevertheless, as they all said, "You just do—if you're human, you do"; "you can't help it."

---

9. Abel and Nelson (2001, p. 29).

Perhaps this is the biggest difference between care in the private and public spheres. In families, people take on caregiving out of necessity and love. They may not want to become primary caregivers, but when circumstances arise, they let themselves be drafted into the role out of sheer loyalty. In agencies and institutions, caregiving is a job. For many caregiving professionals, however, it quickly turns into a labor of love. In a caring community, the overseers of care for the elderly and the infirm would make room for love. To paraphrase Robert Frost, a caring community would be a place where someone not only has to take you in but also has a chance to love you.

References

Abel, Emily. 2001. *Hearts of Wisdom*. Harvard University Press.

Abel, Emily K., and Margaret K. Nelson. 2001. "Intimate Care for Hire." *American Prospect* (May 21): 26–29.

Arno, Peter, Carole Levine, and Margaret Memmott. 2000. "The Economic Value of Informal Caregiving." *Health Affairs* 18 (2): 182–88.

Lipsky, Michael. 1988. *Street-Level Bureaucracy*. Russell Sage Foundation.

Reich, Robert. 1998. *Work of Nations*. Knopf.

Stone, Deborah. 2000a. "Caring by the Book." In *Care Work: Gender, Labor, and the Welfare State*, edited by Madonna Harrington Meyer, 89–111, 315–17. Routledge.

———. 2000b. *Reframing Home Health Care Policy*. Cambridge, Mass.: Radcliffe Public Policy Center.

18

Meeting Tomorrow's Need for Chronic and Long-Term Care

Charles J. Fahey

So MANY VARIABLES affect the need for long-term care and the response to that need that it is virtually impossible to predict what the future holds in store in that area. However, this paper reflects what I feel are the factors that will contribute to that future and posits some desirable elements of it.

The use of the term *long-term care* itself may be both misleading and constraining. Long-term care addresses the reality of loss and how individuals, those close to them, and society as a whole deal with it. This loss is a sometimes gradual, sometimes dramatic degradation of physiological, intellectual, and social capacity that requires substantial and costly support. This loss and the need that accompanies it have become so pervasive that a period of frailty can now be characterized as a predictable part of the human journey. The virtual universality in the human journey of greater or lesser frailty, with its associated costs to individuals, families, and society, makes it a matter of public concern. It may therefore be useful to consider frailty as the overarching concept in the debate over the provision of long-term care.

Frailty as an Organizing Principle

In its context as an organizing principle in the long-term-care discussion, frailty is both a state of being and a process. It involves functional, social, and economic considerations. Central to the concept are the challenges to a person's ability to deal with activities of daily living, insults both minor and devastating, and change. Frailty is likely to be progressive, with some periods of remission, and will ultimately result in the need for care and, finally, in death.

The author acknowledges with gratitude the assistance of Daniel Fox, president of the Milbank Memorial Fund, in the development of many of the ideas expressed here.

Frailty is not easily defined, but it is easily recognized. It manifests itself in many diverse ways that often coalesce into substantial dependence. It may occur as a result of a cataclysmic physical event such as a stroke, a social event such as the loss of a significant other, or an economic event such as the loss of personal savings. In some instances, frailty occurs over time with various individual physical events; in other instances, it is brought on by a sudden cascading of events that can best be characterized as system degradation or failure. The common characteristic of frailty is the loss of the capacity to manage without assistance.

The impact of the increase in the incidence and prevalence of frailty is both personal and social, involving the person, those significant to him or her, and society as a whole. Everyone is at multiple risk, whether as a potential user, a caregiver, or a payer. Typically, increased frailty occurs in the latter part of life, when one's material and social assets may be diminished and income reduced to the minimum for all but the most affluent. Simultaneously, the costs associated with pharmacological agents, new environmental arrangements, and prosthetic devices increase.

Frailty is hard to objectify. It involves endogenous and exogenous factors. Culture, values, psychological strength, and personal financial assets all have an impact on a person's ability to cope with decreased physical capacity. Where one lives, the configuration of one's home, and the willingness of others to help are also significant. Whatever the cause, the frail person has difficulty dealing with the basics of life and manages to do so only at economic, social, and psychological costs.

Current policy tends to implement long-term care that is a step down from care for acute illness. Each intervention for long-term care is built on a medical model, with all of its trappings, but much of the problem actually lies with and calls for social, economic, and environmental approaches with medical add-ons. Unless and until the basic problem is better defined, the foundation of long-term care will be dominated by the culture of illness and disease.

In addition to the historic long-term-care system that is the result of a devolution in acute medical and long-term psychiatric care, the cultural divide evident in virtually all developed countries between health care as a general public responsibility and social care as a personal and welfare function further skews the long-term-care system. Western democracies, with the exception of the United States, have universal entitlements in the area of acute-health-care problems. However, virtually all Western democracies means-test or localize social support and the care of the frail.

Because care of the frail can be costly both to individuals and to state governments, these payers have made extensive use of the bank robber Willy Sutton's principle, "Go where the money is." Medicaid, a part of the compromise that also brought about Medicare, was designed for the medically indigent. It was gradually expanded at the state level to cover care not only for the very sick but also for the frail. Medicare Extended Care Benefits (Part B) were intended to provide a substitute for inpatient hospital days. Over the years, Part B expanded to meet the needs of the frail, only to be contracted for fiscal reasons.

The dominant desires of persons with handicapping conditions are normalcy, activity, and participation. The Americans with Disabilities Act, the *Olmstead* decision, and vibrant advocacy activity are indications of these desires and, to some extent, have moved society to foster inclusiveness as well as, where needed, care programs and facilities that maximize independence and consumer direction. These examples demonstrate the ability of empowered consumers to bring about cultural and systemic changes.

Analogously, various court decisions such as the Willowbrook Consent Decree and effective advocacy on the part of the Association for Retarded Citizens have changed public policy toward frailty. The large institutional approach has given way to smaller, more homelike neighborhood settings for those in need of residential care. The medical component has become secondary, no longer dictating the matrix for the care of the developmentally disabled. This, too, is an example of cultural and structural change resulting from strong and effective, albeit surrogate, consumer advocacy.

The high point of physiological capacity occurs during the ordinary reproductive phase of the life cycle. This is true of all plants and animals, including human beings. After this period, physiological capacity gradually but inexorably declines, with death being the end point. Many compensations can be utilized, however, to mitigate somewhat the decline and its consequences. Moreover, the human executive functions—living responsibly and ethically, developing wisdom, making contributions to society—often increase.

Whether the incidence and prevalence of actual dependency are decreasing is yet to be settled. It is clear that many medical advances are warding off premature death, and numerous pharmacological, prosthetic, and life-style interventions are currently available that can mitigate the likelihood of dependency, though not the underlying potential for frailty, current or future.

Dealing with frailty is as complex as its etiology. Compensations, compromises, and avoidance of potential risks are part of the aging process. Early in the progression, the individual and his or her significant other engage in these strategies more or less successfully but always at a cost—often an escalating one. In this phase, the culture of care is largely what the culture of the individuals and their means allows or dictates. If frailty increases in intensity, the question of personal resources becomes determinative. People of means continue to make choices within the context of their values and the marketplace's response to the value judgments of purchasers. Assisted-living and continuing-care residential facilities and home care are interventions of choice. For those without sufficient means, the options lie within publicly subsidized programs that are largely institutional, highly regulated for safety, and intensely medicalized.

Two overlapping types of aging frailty are particularly challenging: that involving a physical cause and that involving dementia. Often they coexist to a greater or lesser degree, but the care for each condition, at least in the extremes, is quite different. Physical frailty affords greater interpersonal communication and self-direction than dementia. The mixture of the two is at best a challenge for caregivers, as the tendency is to attend to those with little communication and self-direction capacity at the expense of the physically frail.

Chronic and End-of-Life Care

Virtually all older persons develop chronic (that is, persistent and noncorrectable) conditions. In many instances, these problems do not cause a person to be dependent on others, save for skilled medical practitioners who are able to prescribe and monitor life-style factors, pharmacological therapies, and prosthetic devices. However, certain conditions limit a person's capacity to manage without hands-on assistance and will ultimately be the cause of death. Chronic illness is a medical condition. Dependency may or may not be associated with it. When it is, there must be a balance between social and medical concerns, especially if the condition leads to the need for alternate living arrangements.

All persons will die, but the proximity of death, on average, increases with age and frailty. In the developed countries, death from disease has given way to various manifestations of organ deterioration. Despite our limited ability to predict with accuracy the likely time of death, even in the face of serious illness, Medicare will pay for hospice service only for those whose death is expected within six months. Palliative care focuses on those persons whose conditions are not remediable and is geared toward relieving pain and suffering rather than toward cure.

Those receiving chronic-care and hospice services are likely to be the recipients of long-term care and are certainly frail. However, the converse is not true. Many persons who are frail receive neither.

Thoughts on Reform

It is ironic that at a moment of relative affluence, there is little civic dialogue about a societal approach to long-term care and the culture that informs it.

Despite pressing problems inherent in all facets of long-term care, we are in the lull before the storm. We are missing the opportunity for structural reform.

Calls for change exhibit elements of time and intensity, generally related to persons connected with frailty and its impact. The more immediately and intimately people are involved in frailty and long-term care, the more they see the need for reform. Some are keenly aware of the impending crisis but seem unable to put forward an agenda or mobilize a movement that will bring systemic change. Society in general seems to suffer from mass denial, indifference, inertia, and ignorance.

Current long-term-care policy is segmented, incomplete, and often occasioned by bitter exchanges among advocates for various aspects of the system. Focus tends to be upon short-term fixes to relieve the pain experienced by users and fiscal and regulatory concerns of and about providers. There is no agreed-upon civic agenda, yet such an agenda is essential to reform of a system that appears to be both unsustainable and inhumane in its current form.

Strategies toward reform and culture change must take into account immediate issues as well as long-range concerns. Can an approach be fashioned that will enable individuals to cope with the services, setting, and costs associated with dependency? Such policies not only must meet the needs of individuals but also must be sustainable in the light of other legitimate but competing societal needs.

Unless there are dramatic breakthroughs, as yet unforeseen, costs will inevitably escalate for individuals and for society as a whole. Some of the questions that must be addressed are the following:

—What are or should be societal expectations about the responsibility of significant others in caring for their frail partners, family members, and friends?

—Are these expectations realistic, given changing social structures and personal values?

—Does government have only a residual responsibility to care for those who have no resources with which to compensate for their frailty?

—Should government adopt a social insurance approach that involves lifelong, intergenerational sharing of and paying for risks of frailty?

—Would a policy of tax incentives for the purchase of private insurance generate a response adequate to ensuring that reliance on welfare-type programs would be minimal?

—Should governmental policy emphasize a consumer-directed approach in which individuals have complete control over public dollars designated to meet their needs associated with frailty and dependency?

—What are preferred modes of delivery?

—Should marketplace forces determine modes of delivery exclusively, primarily, moderately, or not at all?

—What are the most effective and humane modes of public management of resources and delivery?

—What is the underlying ideology of public quality assurance?

—What is the most effective means to avoiding abuse of individuals and exploitation of the system?

—What is the appropriate role of various levels of government?

Determinants of the Future

Current long-term-care service and systems are extensive and often capital intensive. Individually and collectively, they constitute a significant inertial force whose course is difficult to alter by reason of its sheer size, presence in communities, and powerful political influence. The long-term-care industry is a major employer, especially of low-income people. Union activity and influence are a growing factor. Change in this field will, in all likelihood, come slowly and with considerable difficulty.

Although there has been an extension of life expectancy in the latter part of the twentieth century, with concomitant growth in relative and absolute numbers of older persons, it is not clear whether there has also been an improvement in the health and vigor of the oldest among us. Respected scholars have concluded that there is a compression of morbidity; others disagree. Whatever the reality, it will significantly affect the long-term-care scene.

The consumer of services is not merely the individual who is frail but also others who have legal, moral, and psychological bonds with them. Frailty is a social event intruding on the space and opportunities of many persons. All in the "network" are consumers of long-term care to a greater or lesser degree.

Two sometimes-overlooked realities about the consumer should be noted. First, whether patient or caregiver, the consumer of chronic-care services is likely to be a woman. The difference in life expectancy correlates with the reality that women are often primary caregivers and, if married, are likely to outlive their husbands by several years. The second "new reality" is the emergence of four-generational families with two of the generations in retirement. Thus the proximate next-generation caregiver is likely to be someone in his or her sixties.

In a normal marketplace, consumer desires dictate the kind of goods and services available. This is only partially true, however, in the market for long-term care. Government is the primary purchaser of long-term-care services, at least to the degree that it dictates who is eligible for subsidies, where they can receive services, and how much it will pay providers. Moreover, only a few providers can offer services exclusively to a nonsubsidized clientele. Thus government eligibility criteria, reimbursement policy, and regulatory activities tend to shape the field and its components.

The probable economic capacity of tomorrow's elders is unlikely to support a more consumer-driven marketplace unless there is reform of federal long-term-care policy, with a shift toward social insurance. Although it is impossible to predict with any degree of certainty what will happen, I feel the following directions are desirable:

—a move toward social insurance, a potential third leg of income security, alongside Social Security and Medicare

—a supplemental private market for long-term-care insurance

—retention of residual welfare benefits

—disability-based benefits

—consumer direction

—a demedicalization system

—provision for care at home and in homelike environments

—a better balance of risk and safety

—decent pay for formal caregivers and relief for primary caregivers

Commentary on Part Five

Comment by Richard Bringewatt

This conference has produced a number of excellent ideas for addressing the current problems faced by people needing chronic care, their families, and their providers. One of my greatest fears, however, is that without a targeted, action-driven agenda, many of these ideas will never reach the people who are most responsible for making public health policy. As a result, I suggest that five principles be adopted for shaping a preferred future in care for chronic illness, given the current health policy environment.

First, the characteristics of chronic illness can be used as the lens through which we understand the making of health policy. Chronic illness is multidimensional, interdependent, disabling, ongoing, and personal. I think it is fair to say that most of us who participated in the conference function primarily out of our individual training and experience, and most of us have a segmented training and experience base. So if we talk about chronic care in a hospital, we use a hospital solution. If we talk about chronic illness in a long-term-care setting, chronic care will mean long-term care. If we are in a physician's office, we talk mostly about disease management.

From a consumer perspective, chronic illness is much bigger than any of these perspectives. Chronic illness is not only about disease but also about function, family, and the ability to maintain a preferred way of life; it is multidimensional. Yet most health policy is focused primarily on the biochemical issues of chronic disease. The medical is separated from the psychosocial, and the acute from the long-term. Each illness is treated one disease at a time, even though more than 63 percent of Medicare beneficiaries have two or more chronic conditions, and most people in later life have multiple chronic conditions.[1]

1. Anderson (2001).

People with chronic conditions are primarily concerned with their functional abilities, but the chronic-care system focuses primarily on their illnesses. Chronic conditions are ongoing, and yet care is financed around insurable events and managed around precipitating events, such as hip fractures, strokes, and indications of high blood pressure. Chronic illness is personal and demands provision of services in the home, and yet sometimes the best policymakers can do is talk about making institutions more homelike. If the issues are viewed through these lenses as public policy is made, public policy will not only be different, it will be better, producing better cost and quality outcomes as well as improved patient satisfaction.

Second, it is critical that the policymaking focus be on developing a business case for chronic illness care. Business incentives drive most American institutions, including those in health care, but there is no business case for the care of chronic illness. The structures and incentives that currently exist do not provide care in the most cost-effective way; they appear to exist primarily to preserve historical institutions that were established in 1965.

To develop a business case for chronic illness care, policymakers have to look primarily at the financial incentives at work in current health policy arrangements. The average payment for the top 20 percent of cases (based on cost) under Medicare Plus Choice financing, for example, is about 50 percent of what it would be under fee-for-service reimbursement. Payment is about two-and-a-half times the fee-for-service equivalent for the bottom 20 percent.[2] The prospective payment system for skilled-nursing facilities or home health care offers few incentives for targeting the high-cost users or preventing, delaying, or minimizing the progression of chronic illness. The fee-for-service system, as it applies to hospitals, provides incentives to avoid the medically complex. Primary-care physicians who specialize in the care of frail, medically complex Medicare beneficiaries are the least well paid, and they have the most complex reporting requirements. If physicians are able to hospitalize their patients, they can get paid for every day of care that the patients are in the hospital. If they try to manage care in an outpatient setting, offer prevention services, work with the families, and seek to avoid hospitalizations, they frequently cannot get paid. The current financial incentives are in all the wrong places.

Third, the focus needs to be shifted from the needs of provider systems that were established in 1965 to the needs of tomorrow. There is no health policy in this country today—only budget policy. As a result, interest groups, whether organized around diseases or around provider industry segments, are all

2. Greenwald (2000).

fighting for their piece of the pie. The basic principles of chronic illness identified above are well known, yet health policy has not developed accordingly. It continues to embrace an antiquated industry structure that is no longer in keeping with the times.

A very different world has evolved with advancements in information technology, pharmacology, and other health sciences. Good decisions, whether in actuarial science or public policy, are not made by looking in the rearview mirror. To escape from the current health policy quagmire, policymakers must look to the future, not to the past. We must establish health policy for the twenty-first century, not budget policy for today.

Fourth, I want to stress the importance of building leadership coalitions for a new national agenda. Current health-care trends suggest that our health policy is in a complacency death spiral. Costs are going up with no end in sight, consumer confidence is going down, and other priorities are taking much needed federal dollars. Yet the United States has a crisis on its hands, a crisis that will be resolved only if the different health sectors can find common ground, with a common vision and commitment to work together to develop a better care system for the chronically ill.

Fifth, as this coalition is being built, we need to target a few realistic short-term policy changes that can leverage a better future over time. In this regard, I would suggest four priority targets for next-stage policy intervention. One is to fortify the financial base for mainstream providers of chronic-care services. Payments to physicians, home-health-care agencies, skilled-nursing homes, and other key Medicare providers will be significantly reduced if budget allocations for them are not restored later this year. If we do not fortify our base, the front lines of care will continue to experience a reduction in work force, problems in maintaining quality, and constraints in developing the capacity to serve a new and different health-care consumer.

In addition to fortifying the base, gaps in the benefit package need to be filled. In this regard, prevention services, a pharmacy benefit, and a care coordination benefit should be at the top of a list of priorities. Another target is defining health status adjustments for the chronically ill. This should be addressed in both Medicare Plus Choice policy and fee-for-service policy. Providers along the spectrum need incentives to target, rather than avoid, high-cost patients. This will involve shifting the application of co-payments and deductibles.

Finally, a blueprint for structural reform is needed, and it is needed now. We cannot afford to do everything all at once, but we must get on with the task of preparing to administer health care in a new and different way. A starting point may be standardized provider participation requirements across care settings, where many people are responsible for serving a single person with a chronic condition as that condition progresses across time, place, and profession. A companion effort may be to restructure care management for people who are dually eligible for Medicare and Medicaid.

More attention should be paid to establishing specialized Medicare Plus Choice plans for serving frail, medically complex Medicare beneficiaries. It may be that managed care is best suited for the high-end, advanced, comorbid, complex-care kinds of problems. Some kind of managed fee-for-service arrangement might be necessary as a companion to this next-stage evolution of managed-care financing. This may include, as a matter of priority, a complex-care supplement for physicians who take care of frail, medically complex Medicare beneficiaries. It may also include the establishment of an episode-of-care payment system for the full array of Medicare benefits associated with an acute episode, such as in the care and treatment of hip fractures and strokes. Bite-sized public policy initiatives such as these are realistic in the short term and make the most sense over the long term.

These are tough times, and tough times demand vision and hard work by a small group of knowledgeable leaders committed to change. We must leave our guns at the door. Policymakers, planners, providers, and consumers need to work together in solving one of the most complex health-care problems of our time. With vision, tenacity, and hard work, we can produce a better world for people with serious and disabling chronic conditions, the largest, highest-cost, and fastest-growing service group in U.S. health care today.

Comment by William Scanlon

The conference on which this volume is based made real progress in a number of areas. At the same time, when I look at the title for this section, "Visions for the Future," I am somewhat troubled. I participated in a similar conference in 1985. At that time, the interest in long-term care was motivated by a desire to prepare for the aging of the baby boomers. I recall expressing some doubts that we had identified the objectives for the long-term-care policy we were trying to formulate. Well, here I am, seventeen years later, still doubtful.

What services should be guaranteed to persons with disabilities? What protections from catastrophe, financial or otherwise, should be afforded? Without some consensus on such fundamental objectives, it is hard to have fruitful discussions on how best to divide responsibility for achieving desired outcomes between the public and private sectors or what mechanisms would help each sector fulfill its role.

Identifying our objectives will be critical to making real progress in developing long-term-care policy that addresses the impending challenges. That process would be facilitated somewhat if we had a clearer consensus on what we are talking about. There is a language problem in discussions on long-term care. Words have different meanings depending on the speaker and the listener. Agreement at the outset on the nature of long-term care would be helpful, and I would like to offer some thoughts in that regard.

Our current health insurance programs have considerable potential to treat and manage chronic illness (for example, diabetes, renal disease, chronic obstructive pulmonary disease). Care of chronic illnesses doubtlessly could be improved, but those improvements are feasible within the context of the existing health care system. However, those programs currently available have limited capacity to assist with disability.

Our focus when we talk of long-term care should be the care and assistance people need to maintain their life-styles in the face of disability. (In talking about long-term care, I prefer to use the term *life-style,* rather than *life,* to reinforce the distinction from other health services. In addition, while these services may be essential to maintaining life, how they are delivered and where—the setting—are elements related to life-style.) Long-term care is not a health service that is designed to improve a condition or to prevent deterioration in a chronic condition. Too often we confuse long-term care with health services aimed at maintaining health status. This confusion does disservice to the services involved in long-term care.

Early on in the research on long-term care, when we were trying to measure the benefits of home care, people were disappointed because the care patients received did not result in functional improvements in their activities of daily living. Long-term care is not aimed at changing a disability that may be permanent and may also be worsening. It is about preparing meals, getting dressed, bathing, and going to the toilet—assistance that compensates for disability to allow patients to maintain their life-styles.

Moreover, the need for long-term care before we die, particularly extensive formal long-term care, is a risk, not a certainty. There is a danger in drawing attention to the burden long-term care may involve and the importance of preparing for it that the risk will be grossly exaggerated; in fact, a relatively small fraction of the population will be significantly affected. Saving in anticipation of one's long-term-care need is not the most rational approach. Too many individuals would die without experiencing the need for extensive long-term care but having forgone the benefits of using the resources set aside for long-term care for other purposes. From an economic perspective, it makes more sense to insure against the risk of needing long-term care; we need mechanisms that allow us to share our risk with others.

At this point, however, not many people can spread much of their risk. The only widespread insurance comes through the Medicaid program. However, Medicaid is, in effect, insurance against further catastrophe—once you have had the catastrophic experience of being bankrupted by long-term care expenses. Medicaid then provides protection against not getting services in the future. We have had about twenty years of growing attention paid to private long-term-care insurance as a way of providing more protection against risk. Yet few people have such a policy, and it is uncertain how much many such policies will cover.

Mark Warshawsky's proposal involves the type of innovative thinking that we need to explore, to find ways to make greater risk protection available. It addresses two fundamental problems with today's private long-term-care insurance market: the unaffordability of long-term-care insurance and its lack of appeal to a large share of the population. Because of extensive underwriting practices, people who are at high risk of needing services have great difficulty in purchasing long-term care policies; and the "good risks" do not want to pay the higher premiums that would follow if the "bad risks" were included in their risk pool. Finding a way to weaken this disincentive for the good risks is a potentially effective way of broadening the number of persons who could be covered. In addition, the limited sales of long-term-care insurance policies now are not the result of a dearth of offerings. Rather, there seems to be limited interest in stand-alone policies. Packaging long-term-care insurance with other financial products may be an effective means of sparking greater interest and further broadening coverage.

Even if the private long-term-care insurance market begins to grow rapidly, the public sector will retain a significant role in financing long-term care. Insurance will still be beyond the reach of two groups of people: those who cannot afford insurance policies that address their needs and those whose purchased insurance proves inadequate to their needs. The two groups that Monsignor Fahey mentions are examples—people born with a need that is going to continue throughout their life span and people who at a young age acquire a disability and are going to need continuing support; in both cases, because of good medical care, their needs could last decades.

A review of the programs offered in the fifty states shows significant variation in the extent of public support and the types of services being provided. What is sorely missing is knowledge of the effects. What are the consequences of different levels and types of support for the individuals who are getting care? What are the consequences for families who play a key role in providing supplementary, or often all, care? Without some understanding of those consequences, there is no way to evaluate alternative approaches and to be able to choose among them as to what we would like to pursue on a more widespread basis.

Cost-effectiveness is not and should never have been the measure in selecting among alternatives. Relative costs are not the only relevant consideration; and the alternatives are not comparable. We need to focus on cost-benefit comparisons, but we have to find much better means of defining the benefits associated with assistance. The difficulty is readily apparent in looking at the difference in benefits that may come from receiving the same types of assistance at home or in an institution.

Public policy should not be a barrier to creating caring communities. There are, however, other significant barriers to accomplishing that goal. Medicare home health care is a great example of the difficulties encountered in trying to provide a publicly managed service benefit in long-term care. Before 1997, Medicare offered a literal blank check to home-health-care agencies to use in providing as many services as they chose to beneficiaries. There was virtually no accountability—fewer than 1 percent of claims were ever reviewed. The result was, overall, dramatic growth in the use of services. What is disturbing is that growth followed no pattern that seemed related to meeting beneficiaries' needs. In some states there was no growth at all over the early 1990s; in others, the increase in the use of services was extremely high. In 1997 a Medicare user of home health care in Maryland received, on average, about 35 visits during the course of the year. An average home-based Medicare recipient in Louisiana, on average, received about 150 visits.

In looking at the variation in use across states, the only correlate that we could find was the for-profit proportion of the industry in each state. When large shares of the industry in a state operated for profit, services were used more often; and the nonprofit Visiting Nurse Associations provided more care than in other states. This is the kind of response to incentives one might expect, but it is also the kind of response that creates a strong sense that resources are not being spent appropriately and that a change in policy is needed to gain some control.

In response, the 1997 Balanced Budget Act eliminated the blank check to Medicare and created first an interim payment system and then a prospective payment system for home health care. The experience under these systems has not created a caring community; rather, it reflects the economic incentives in these payment systems. There is no question that the interim payment system, in place from 1997 through 2000, was flawed in the new restrictions it imposed on payment for home-based health care. At the same time, agencies' responses to the system were not totally dictated by the elements of the system. Services were reduced much more than the system required. Beneficiaries were sometimes told, "Medicare will not allow it," when in fact Medicare would allow and would pay for at least some of the services that were being discussed.

Beginning in 2000, the prospective payment system replaced the flawed interim payment system. Unfortunately, it too is potentially flawed. It simply reflects the average service delivery of the period before the Balanced Budget Act, without assurance that earlier levels of service were too low or too high. It makes lump-sum payments for sixty days of care—payments that range from $1,100 to $6,000 for one of these sixty-day episodes of care; but there is no definition of what an episode of care should entail. What services should a beneficiary receive? It requires only that a beneficiary receive five visits in those sixty days; there is no further definition of what constitutes adequate services. The immediate concern is the system's inherent incentive to reduce the care provided and the absence of any countervailing mechanism to ensure accountability for appropriate care. Once again, services can be inappropriately denied on grounds that "Medicare will not allow it."

Finally, one important element in improving the financing and delivery of services is enhancement of the position of aides, who provide most of the services to people with disabilities. Increasing wages and job satisfaction would undoubtedly attract more individuals to these positions, but it will not be enough. The demographics of the baby boomers and the generations that follow them are such that there will not be enough members of the working-age population to provide care in the manner that we do today. The numbers are simply not there.

We need to begin thinking about how to enhance the productivity of long-term-care workers and to find ways to provide some services without labor at all. How can we use equipment to greater benefit? How can we create group settings, which can have real economics of scale, that are more attractive as homes for people needing care? In other words, how can we use capital to improve care delivery? We may have a nursing shortage today; but looking to 2030, the potential problem is magnified many times.

References

Anderson, Gerard. 2001. "Fact Sheet on 'Multiple Chronic Conditions Complicate Care and Treatment.'" Baltimore: Partnership for Solutions (December).

Greenwald, Leslie. 2000. "Overview of Risk Adjustment for Medicare + Choice." Paper prepared for Risk Assessment and Risk Adjustment for People with Disabilities: A Technical Conference. National Research Hospital Center for Health and Disability Research, Rosslyn, Virginia, November 17, 2000.

Epilogue

19

National Policymakers on Long-Term-Care Policy

Remarks by Benjamin Cardin

Since September 11, 2001, Congress has been consumed by the defense of our country and dealing with the aftermath of the terrorist attacks. I have never seen any event unify our nation more than what happened that day. For a short period of time, at least, we were not partisans in Washington, we were working together on the same team.

The nation set four basic priorities as a result of the attacks on our country, and I think we have done a good job at attaining them. The first was to take care of the people who were directly affected, the families and the businesses, and Congress responded by opening up our hearts and our resources. We passed a bill to aid the airline industry, and we are in the process of passing a bill to aid the insurance industry.

Our second major priority was to defend this country. We established a separate department for homeland security. We have changed our entire approach to national security. Public health priorities have changed to make this nation safer for all of us. Our third priority was to go after those who attacked our country, and our president and our military have done a superb job.

In Afghanistan and throughout the world, in more than seventy nations, we have exercised our diplomatic and economic rights to deal with those who support terrorism. Our fourth priority is probably the most challenging, and that is to get back to some form of normalcy in this country. That has been tough.

Congress is trying to do its part. Partisan battles are back, so we are starting to return to a more normal environment.

The surplus, which was projected last year to be $5.6 trillion over a ten-year period, is now projected to be $1.6 trillion, a loss of $4 trillion in one year. A lot of this is attributable to erroneous projections. Some estimates from the Office of Management and Budget make Enron look like a model of responsible accounting. So we have had some problems in the way we do our forecasting. The point is, though, that as we start debating how to stimulate our economy, whether to enact additional tax cuts, how to prepare our nation for homeland security, and what we are going to do to protect our transportation systems, we also must debate what we are going to do to strengthen the Medicare program and to improve the long-term-care system in this country.

It is time for us to take a closer look at what we are doing with social insurance here in the United States, to look at the graying of America. One hundred years ago the average life expectancy was 47. Now it is 80. The elderly population (over 65 years of age) in the United States in 2030 is projected to be 70 million, twice the number in 1997.

In March, 2002, we marked the twelfth anniversary of the Pepper Commission. That commission was my initiation into the Ways and Means Committee in Congress and my involvement in social insurance programs. Claude Pepper, of course, was the champion of the elderly, and a hero to me. There was a lot of talk about the Pepper Commission's report but very little action.

The time has come for us to modernize our social insurance programs to fulfill the needs of elderly and disabled Americans. The current situation is unacceptable. Medicare today covers only 53 percent of our seniors' health-care costs. If you ask most Americans about seniors' access to health care, they will reply, "Oh, they're doing great, they have Medicare. Seniors are the only age group of Americans that is guaranteed health insurance coverage."

That impression misses most of the story: Medicare notwithstanding, seniors have the highest out-of-pocket costs for health care of any age group. This is not a statistic we should be proud of. Medicare does not provide much protection at all for the day-to-day long-term-care needs and nursing care for our senior population. Medicaid is an option, but do we really want to tell our seniors that they have to go into poverty to qualify for coverage?

Medicaid is not social insurance. It is welfare. Our seniors think it is social insurance; they think it is their insurance program. They think they are entitled to it as a matter of right. Medicaid is a program for the poor; eligibility is determined by level of income and assets. Our seniors deserve a better approach to long-term care.

In nursing care, the trend has been to try to encourage personal responsibility by promoting private long-term-care insurance for nursing-home care. I think that makes some sense. If I were designing a program today for nursing care for our population—and many persons who need long-term care are under 65—I would encourage people to buy some long-term-care insurance. It would be affordable, it would be a known risk, and the Medicare program could take care of any uncovered expenses. Those who have major needs would be covered by the social insurance program, and those who could not afford private insurance would be covered by Medicaid. This would actually cost the government less money, not more. The problem is in coordinating the various levels of government—Medicaid being a federal program administered by the states, and Medicare a strictly federal program—and the funding coming from several sources: payroll taxes, premiums, and general support from the taxpayers.

Congress has not been able to figure out through its budget rules and intergovernmental rules how to combine these funding sources to create a rational system for financing nursing care in this country. Encouraging more private insurance, changing the Medicare system, and working with the revenue-sharing systems of our local governments so that we capture the money that is available to fund a more rational system of nursing-care financing are promising directions.

Congress took a small step in that direction in 2000, when President Bill Clinton signed legislation that would enable federal employees to purchase long-term-care insurance at group rates. The U.S. Office of Personnel Management will be offering these plans in March. The plans are not subsidized, but they are much more affordable than policies offered in the individual market. The number of federal workers who will take advantage of the program is not yet known; we would probably see higher participation levels if we created incentives within government insurance programs.

Institutional nursing care is not the major long-term-care focus of Medicare. Home health care is a much more significant part of the long-term-care commitment in our Medicare program, and it has worked fairly well. However, the Balanced Budget Act of 1997 made changes in Medicare's reimbursement structure that had nothing to do with health policy and everything to do with hitting specific budget targets. So in 1999, Congress based cost reimbursement on 1994 data. That hurt us in Maryland, where we happened to have a cost-effective home-health-care system at the time. We were, in effect, penalized by the base that was used, and we were reimbursed less than higher-cost, less efficient states. In Louisiana, for example, where the average costs for each beneficiary were much higher in 1994, Medicare recipients were in better shape. That approach was unfair, and we are still trying to recover from it today. We have made some improvements in the past two years, but a 15 percent cut is scheduled to go into effect on October 1, 2002, if a Medicare bill is not enacted and signed by the president sometime this year.

Rehabilitative therapy services fall into the same category. Physical, occupational, and speech therapists treat some of our most vulnerable patients:

people who have had strokes, those who are recovering from hip replacements, and ALS (amyotrophic lateral sclerosis, often called Lou Gehrig's disease) patients all need rehabilitation therapy. The Balanced Budget Act, however, placed annual caps of $1,500 on reimbursement for rehabilitative therapies. No one seems to know how this figure was derived; and no one on Capitol Hill can defend this approach. Too often, our nation's social insurance policies are driven by budgets rather than by right policy. Since 1997, Congress has placed moratoriums on application of the therapy caps, but they will be imposed if we are unable to pass a Medicare bill by the end of this year.

I want to compliment the Centers for Medicare and Medicaid Services' administrator, Tom Scully, and Tommy Thompson, the secretary of the Department of Health and Human Services, for moving forward on quality issues in long-term care because it is important to ensure quality as well as provide appropriate reimbursement. We also must not relax the nursing-home regulations. We need to strengthen them, particularly the inspections. I am hopeful that the Bush administration will decide to move in that direction.

The tremendous shortage in nursing personnel also needs to be addressed. I have introduced legislation for the past several years aimed at the financing of graduate medical education. It does not make much sense to pay for training costs through Medicare's rate structure, and we still do that for our resident physicians. We need to have a reliable source of training for our medical personnel, including nurses and allied health professionals. The need for nursing schools is especially acute. In my own state, we have reduced nurse training, mainly because of cost, not because of the economics of nursing; but the decrease in qualified nursing staff has been a cost to the state. We have got to figure out a better way, and the federal government has a major role to play here.

Assisted living is an issue that receives little attention in Washington, though it is probably the issue of greatest concern to my constituents. Many of my constituents do not need nursing care but are consigned to nursing homes either because they can get Medicare reimbursement for the assistance they need or because they have no family members who can care for them. The options are limited; and the nursing home—the most expensive of the options—is frequently chosen simply because its expenses are reimbursable.

Many seniors would much prefer to be in assisted-living facilities. The main barrier to access is unaffordability. Most assisted living today is paid for out of the residents' private funds. We have made progress in the Medicaid program by allowing the services to be reimbursable for very-low-income seniors. We have made some progress at the U.S. Department of Housing and Urban Development (HUD) by allowing Section 8 vouchers to be used for the rent portion of assisted living, but the program is not yet ready to be put into operation. We do have a demonstration program in Maryland that is using Medicaid and HUD funds in an effort to provide some assisted-living opportunities for low- and moderate-income seniors, but as a nation, we still have not developed a way to combine health care and housing—a pressing need for many seniors.

This is not just a question of financing, it is also a question of quality. The number of assisted-living facilities in this country has doubled in the past seven years. What concerns me a great deal is that often people going into these homes know very little about procedures: What will happen if their current physical condition deteriorates? What are the requirements for living in the home? What services will be provided? One of the jobs of government is to provide legitimate protections to its citizens where needed; but there is no clear definition of assisted living in this country, and government has not taken on this issue of standards and procedures in assisted-living facilities.

The 1997 Balanced Budget Act was not all bad: it did establish, for the first time, preventive services for seniors within Medicare. I was involved in that initiative with Representative Bill Thomas, who was chairman of the House Ways and Means Committee's Subcommittee on Health at the time. We worked on a preventive health-care measure that ultimately became law. It was a good bill. It provides for bone density testing for osteoporosis, mammograms without deductibles, prostate screening, colorectal screenings, pap smears, cervical exams, and diabetes self-management. Congress deemed these services important enough to include them as basic benefits within the Medicare system for all seniors. If we really want to create a cost-effective health system in this country, then we should encourage more preventive health-care services.

There is one glaring absence in the Medicare program: prescription medicines. They keep people well. How many people would select an insurance plan that did not include prescription drug coverage? Medicare is the only "insurance plan" that lacks such coverage—and seniors are most in need of prescription drug coverage.

Prescription drugs help patients manage their diseases. Without the medicines, they are likely to need more intensive and expensive health care, which, in the case of seniors, will be paid for courtesy of the government. That makes very little sense. I understand why a prescription medicine benefit was not included in the original Medicare legislation in 1965. It was not a feature of most private health plans at the time; medications were not as expensive as they are now; and far fewer drugs were available for outpatient management of disease. Even the dangers of high cholesterol were unknown back then.

But medicine has changed. Many diseases can be controlled through medication. The problem is that prescription drugs are very expensive. In many cases, we are talking about maintenance: patients will be taking them for the rest of their lives; they cannot change the dosage; they will need to take the full pill every day. Seniors are making trade-offs in their use of limited financial resources because their medications are so expensive.

So I favor including prescription medicines within the Medicare system, and I have devised legislation that leads us in that direction. It is called the Essential Medicines for Medicare Act. Comprehensive coverage will entail huge costs to the insurance program—not to society, because we are incurring these expenses anyway. So rather than doing it all at one time, we could select the prescriptions covered on a cost-benefit basis: diabetes, hypertension, congestive heart disease, major depression, and rheumatoid arthritis can all be more or less effectively managed by prescription drugs, thereby avoiding hospitalization. These medicines are not a matter of choice; taking them can mean the difference between successful outpatient management of a disease and complex treatment in a hospital; in the extreme case, it can be a matter of life and death.

Diabetes, for example, is the leading cause of end-stage renal disease. A diabetic is twice as likely as the nondiabetic to suffer from heart disease or a stroke and forty times more likely to have a leg amputated. Each year Medicare pays for fifty-six thousand amputations, at a cost of $700 million annually. Diabetes can be successfully managed with medication; but seniors who do not qualify for Medicaid or other forms of medical assistance and cannot afford to pay for prescribed medications will develop a much more complex medical condition that requires more complicated and far more costly treatment—at government expense. The bill I have introduced proposes coverage of prescription drugs as part of the basic Medicare benefit package, with a $250 deductible, a 20 percent co-payment for brand names, and no co-payment for generics, to encourage their use.

I am not certain what will happen with a prescription drug benefit this year, but the modernization of Medicare will be on the table, and we will certainly be debating the Medicare Plus Choice program. I am a strong believer in additional choices for our seniors, but Medicare Plus Choice, as currently constructed, has failed. I do not know how much more we have to do to demonstrate that it is not working. More than 1 million people have been abandoned by their health maintenance organizations (HMOs). Maryland had eight HMOs available to our seniors in 1997. Today, we have one—and that one has capped enrollment; so seniors have virtually no choice of HMO coverage. The cost to join, of course, is much higher than it was in 1997; in fact, premiums have quadrupled.

What choice of plans does a Maryland senior now have? None. I support encouraging an increase in the private insurance market's interest in Medicare, but why not have a government managed-care option as well? If the private insurance market is not interested, let's have our own. This is not a novel suggestion. The Municipal Health Systems demonstration program, which started before I came to Congress, is still funded in four cities. The largest single demonstration happens to be in the Third Congressional District of Maryland—my district—and in that program, Medicare pays a little more than it would for traditional fee-for-service coverage.

The program uses the existing public health system to serve low-income seniors. It provides prescription drug coverage and other preventive health-care services, and it manages the care of enrollees. The seniors are in an HMO for all intents and purposes. And it is working. It is saving the government money. This program should be used as a model to provide more options to our seniors.

It is time to rework our social insurance programs for long-term care. The major stumbling block will be the budget issues we are presently confronting. Because Medicare is a federal insurance program and Medicaid is a federal and state program, reimbursement flows pose significant problems. The U.S program for low-income housing is also a federal program, with a lot of private money and some local money, but it has managed to overcome some of these disbursement problems. It is difficult to capture all the funding sources in this current climate, but we could do a much better job of it.

Congress needs new ideas, and some of the old ideas need to be reworded and presented again. Many members of Congress—on both sides of the aisle—want us to come up with a better system than we have today. We are certainly proud of our record on social insurance in this country. Medicare and Social Security have been tremendous programs.

Thanks to social insurance programs, seniors today are less likely than any other age group of Americans to be living in poverty; they are certainly better off than children. We can do better, however, and we know that health care costs are going to continue to increase. Housing costs will continue to increase much faster than inflation, and we need to figure out a way to meet seniors' needs in a cost-effective way. I thank the conference participants for their contributions thus far and look forward to working with them in addressing the needs of our senior citizens.

Remarks by Thomas A. Scully

The Centers for Medicare and Medicaid Services (CMS), of which I am the administrator, employs more than forty-six hundred people, including more than a thousand employees in ten regional offices, and has a budget of $254 billion. Because of its sheer size, it moves slowly. Moreover, the agency does not really run the programs; contractors run the programs—at present, fifty-one contractors, most of which provide coverage under Blue Cross. As well intentioned as these contractors are, ours is an unwieldy system, and contract reform is high on the CMS reform agenda. In addition, there are thirty thousand State Children's Health Insurance Program (SCHIP) staff. Our people know the frustration of the health-care community—physicians, hospitals, and others—in trying to get answers from Washington or Baltimore.

Tommy Thompson, the secretary of the Department of Health and Human Services, is the driving force behind the agency reforms. Issues that hold a prominent place on the reform agenda include expanded access to health insurance for the poor, provision and financing of long-term care for the elderly, prescription medicine coverage, and improvement in the responsiveness of the agency to the customers and providers it serves.

Expanded Coverage

A lot of our long-term-care problems are related to the way long-term care is financed. The options most people use at the moment are strictly limited: Medicaid, Medicare, and private pay. Long-term-care insurance is another option, but at present few people carry it. There appears to be bipartisan support for proposals that would encourage consumers to buy long-term-care insurance when they turn 62. Tax incentives to do so will go a long way toward increasing participation; there are currently no such incentives in the tax code. The system as it stands, which requires seniors to spend down their assets so that Medicaid will pay their nursing-home expenses, is neither good social policy nor good fiscal policy.

People need to begin to prepare for the risk of needing long-term care while they are in their middle years, as part of their overall financial planning. From an actuary's point of view, it makes no sense to start buying insurance at the age of 65 for a predictable event that is likely to happen when the insured is 75: the premium would be beyond most people's reach. Long-term-care insurance is high on the reform agenda—it probably should have received attention twenty years ago. Until we start thinking about the financing mechanisms to pay for long-term care and get people to start thinking about their long-term-care financing options, many of the problems will persist.

Access to health insurance for low-income people is another important issue. In his 2001 budget, President George W. Bush proposed a significant refundable tax credit for the purchase of health insurance. Refundable tax credits are sometimes misunderstood by the public. Some look at them as "welfare for the rich." In fact, the opposite is true: refundable tax credits go only to the poor. They are, in effect, a negative income tax. A person who qualifies for the credit is refunded—in the form of a reduction in tax owed or as a cash reimbursement—the amount of the credit. The refundable tax credit is the least bureaucratic and most effective way to subsidize insurance for low-income people and reduce the number of uninsured—42 million, at last count (2001).

The president's proposal gave $1,000 for each qualifying low-income person or $2,000 for each qualifying low-income family in tax credits toward purchase of a Blue Cross policy. The sum is given to a certified insurance company as a transfer payment from the Department of the Treasury. Some members of Congress would prefer to see access to insurance for low-income families provided through Medicaid and SCHIP. The debate is understandable, but it has continued for fifteen years, and until the president's proposal not much progress had been made.

The proposal got little attention in 2001. The attacks of September 11 displaced most other items on the national agenda. The 2002 Congress, when it reconvenes, will, I hope, get back into serious debate about access, especially as it relates to long-term care. People who lack insurance coverage get access to health care through emergency rooms, and they have a lot more chronic long-term problems. A mechanism to insure them satisfies the requirements of good social policy as well as good fiscal policy.

We also need to start thinking about creating disease-specific demonstrations. Mississippi Delta residents, for example, have triple the national rate of diabetes, quadruple the rate of heart attacks, and triple the rate of strokes. Diet is part of the problem: fried catfish is a far more popular menu item in the Delta than steamed broccoli. Disease management programs hold great promise for healing both medical and budgetary ills. We need to encourage local health-care delivery systems to take the long view and provide comprehensive disease-specific programs for diabetes, stroke, heart attacks, and a variety of other illnesses in which life-style factors play a part.

The Program of All-Inclusive Care for the Elderly (PACE) is a joint Medicare-Medicaid program for dual eligibles that merges state and federal funds to pay for day care and intensive home-health-care services to the elderly, thereby keeping them out of nursing homes. Definitive research on the financial impact has not been conducted, but the program is probably more cost-effective for both the states and the federal government. What is certain is that the patients are much happier.

Not all of the states are persuaded that the program is a good idea, however; that may be, in part, because of the limited number of demonstrations that have been conducted. Medicaid is a complicated program, and some state directors may either be unaware of or not understand the PACE demonstration. Anyone who has seen the program in operation, however, wants to get a PACE program up and running, The Centers for Medicare and Medicaid Services will quickly approve all requests for the program because we have only a handful of them around the country. They should be energetically promoted.

Disease management is sometimes a better alternative than managed care. ElderCare offers comprehensive nursing-home care under a capitated defined-benefits plan. Both the ElderCare and PACE models have had great success and hold much promise.

Prescription Medications

Medicare prescription drug reform is another important issue. The government has been divided over the form it should take: the Bush administration prefers the Breaux-Frist model, whereby seniors' prescription medications are paid for only in a capitated reformed Medicare program, whereas the Democrats have been arguing for a fee-for-service drug benefit within the current fee-for-service program. In late July 2001, however, just before Congress left Washington for the summer break, President Bush made an effort at compromise, offering to split the difference: he agreed to accept a new Medicare fee-for-service plan that would include a drug benefit, but not along the lines of the existing Part A, Part B deductible system. Under the present system, most seniors buy Medigap insurance, which provides first-dollar coverage, and consequently they tend to be insensitive to cost.

President Bush proposed a reform of Medigap, with reasonable co-payments and reasonable deductibles, for the nonpoor. The Part A and Part B deductibles would be combined, and the Medicare fee-for-service program modernized. A fee-for-service drug benefit would be included.

The president announced his proposal shortly before the August recess. Congress resumed just before the September 11 attacks, and the issue faded from view. I hope that, when the debate resumes, the proposal will be given serious consideration.

To those who argue that the changes are too much to ask for in an election year, I reply that no year is easy. The president's proposal is not a drug benefit, but it is a momentum-building first step toward a drug benefit. Seniors will not be happy with it. Even if Congress were to pass Senator Bob Graham's bill or Representative Bill Thomas's bill tomorrow, it would take three or four years to get a prescription drug benefit up and running. The common denominator of the two bills is that both are based on pharmacy benefits management models and aim at consolidating seniors into large purchasing groups.

Any such drug benefit will be administered by the Centers for Medicare and Medicaid Services, and we have as yet no idea how to pay pharmacists at the point of sale and no experience in running a drug benefit. We ought at least to get seniors in pools of four hundred thousand or five hundred thousand to start buying drugs at a relative market discount, as Blue Cross and other health insurance plans do.

Consumer Education

Over the past decade or two, the nursing-home industry has had significant problems with quality of care; even if the industry is fixing those problems, there are still enormous perception problems. The quality of care in nursing homes can be investigated in a number of ways, but I am an advocate of outcomes-based measurement standards. When my office began researching ways to improve nursing-home care, I approached the nursing homes, the care workers' unions, and patient advocacy groups to invite their participation. To their credit, they all were eager to work with us. At the suggestion of some patient advocate groups, we put together a quality measurement initiative based somewhat on the end-stage renal disease (ESRD) model.

End-stage renal disease is the extreme form of diabetes. It has a relatively small patient base, but it probably includes our sickest patients, who require the most expensive care, and has the highest percentage of minority patients. End-stage renal disease became our model for a number of reasons: First, the ESRD Medicare payment system is complicated, and payment system is one area in serious need of reform. Second, the many dialysis centers around the country provide excellent treatment of diabetes patients. Third, the CMS already has a large database on ESRD treatment at these centers, which gives us a great ability to track outcomes. Finally, most dialysis beneficiaries are not aware of this database (though it is on our website), so we have a high hurdle to get over in educating beneficiaries about their treatment options—another item on the reform agenda. Roughly 350,000 ESRD beneficiaries are now covered by, or at least eligible for, Medicare.

Nursing homes were selected for our demonstration because we had extensive data on their performance. (We are hoping to inaugurate a similar project for home-health-care providers in the near future.) The Minimum Data Set for Nursing Home Resident Assessment and Care Screening (MDS) has a wealth of raw data on nursing homes. We asked Ken Kaiser and the National Quality

Forum to perform research for us. Ken agreed to select, on a very quick turnaround, a number of quality indicators in nursing homes for our six-state demonstration program.[1] By the spring of 2002, we had data on thirteen identifiable outcomes for every nursing home in those six states. On April 24, and again in November, the data were published in all major newspapers in each state, giving the relative risk-adjusted quality measures of nursing-home outcomes. This demonstration will enable patients in those states to make informed choices about their long-term care.

The demonstration is not intended to be a substitute for survey and certification. Rather, it is a tool for consumers to use in selecting the long-term-care facilities most appropriate to their needs and circumstances. Americans presently can more readily find information on buying a used car than on locating quality nursing-home care.

One problem we have encountered is that many senior beneficiaries do not understand their programs. To correct that problem, the CMS spent $80 million in 2002 on an ad campaign to inform beneficiaries of a toll-free hotline that directs callers to area-specific information on nursing homes, dialysis centers, health plans, and Medigap plans. We ran a large Telemundo/Univision campaign to get the message out to Spanish-speaking seniors. At its peak, the hotline took sixty-five thousand calls a day, and over the course of the program we have averaged about fifty thousand calls a day. People are obviously looking for answers.

Agency Responsiveness

As part of our effort to improve our responsiveness toward beneficiaries and providers alike, the CMS has created eleven open-door policy groups that operate over the telephone. I chair three of them: the rural health group, the nursing-home group, and the long-term-care group. The long-term-care group usually draws a large number of participants, and the rural hospital group often has 150 people on the call. The idea is not to reform the health-care system; nor is it to reinvent the American Hospital Association. We are trying, instead, to address one of the primary frustrations with the Health Care Financing Administration, to create a forum through which legitimate gripes with Medicare or Medicaid, either from consumers or from providers, can be voiced and agency staff can learn what problems need to be fixed. So far, I think it is working.

We aggressively pursue complaints of fraud and abuse. On the other hand, most providers are honest and responsible, and through the open-door groups the CMS is trying to improve its relations with providers.

---

1. We had chosen five states; the sixth approached us, imploring us to include it.

In sum, our major reform initiatives at the Centers for Medicare and Medicaid Services at the moment are aimed at educating beneficiaries on their options for care and becoming more responsive to providers and consumers alike. Once these goals have been met, we hope to move on to the issues of expanding coverage to the uninsured and providing seniors with a Medicare drug benefit.

Remarks by Mark McClellan

One of the interesting things about the discussion of long-term-care issues and disability is the truly dynamic nature of the problems it addresses. I mean "dynamic" in two senses. One is that the population itself has become healthier over time. Disability rates have been declining steadily, as has been clearly shown in work by many researchers for a number of years now. According to some of my own research, this reflects, in part, trends in the availability, use, and quality of medical treatment. Medical care, as well as other factors, such as improvements in life-style, socioeconomic status, education, and the like, have been making an important difference in the incidence and burden of disability in our society.

In addition, the treatment of disability when it occurs has changed enormously. I have had the pleasure in recent months of spending a lot of time working with President George Bush's New Freedom Initiative. This is a set of programs in the government that are following the latest round of implementation of activities related to the Americans with Disabilities Act—including the full implementation of the *Olmstead* decision from several years ago—that are focused on encouraging the government to take steps to help people with disabilities participate fully in society. That includes both younger persons with disabilities participating in the work force and older persons who may or may not be retired.

Older persons with disabilities who might otherwise end up in institutions now have a much broader range of options available to help them get the assistance they need in a setting that is more suitable to their preferences, better integrated with their traditional home and family lives, and much more integrated into the community. These are promising directions, and I hope they will continue. We would like to do what we can through federal policies to support disability activities and to support further research that can lead to improvements in disability rates as well as improvements in the treatment and support options available for people with chronic illnesses and disability in the years ahead.

More than 12 million people use some form of long-term care today, the vast majority of them residing in communities and relying as well on unpaid care from family members—particularly wives, daughters, and other women. Despite the trends toward reduced rates of disability and innovative treatments to assist and substitute for personal care for the disabled, it is widely expected that the demands on these caregivers will increase in the years ahead. Although people are living longer and healthier lives, the sheer numbers—a projection of 70 million elderly by 2030—will make this an even more pressing policy problem than it is today.

The needs of this population are increasingly diverse. Whereas some people need and might even prefer institutional assistance, many do not. Moreover, many have disabilities that affect certain activities of daily living but not others, and the treatments available to help them are becoming increasingly diverse.

The options available to provide assistance and support for these activities, however, are remarkably limited. Many people have to rely, first and foremost, on personal savings and family assets. The vital support of family members can be strained by the multiple demands of children, careers, and aging parents.

Thus many people with serious disabilities, particularly at older ages, wind up on Medicaid. Medicaid pays for more than 70 percent of nursing-home days in this country, and despite all of our efforts to shore up alternative options for supporting long-term care, Medicaid's share has not changed much in recent years. Alternative arrangements are needed, to avoid institutionalization wherever possible and to provide options that do not force seniors to "spend down" all of their assets when it is not.

Over the past year, the administration has developed a number of initiatives in this area. One set of options relates to providing more innovative kinds of assistance for lower-income and spend-down populations. The administration is taking steps to increase flexibility in Medicaid programs, to keep those with long-term disabilities who are Medicare beneficiaries, Medicare-Medicaid dual-eligible beneficiaries, or eligible only for Medicaid in the community. We are already working with a number of states to support community- and home-based services as alternatives to institutionalization for Medicaid beneficiaries.

A second important area involves better options to avoid Medicaid spend-down. One of the president's major proposals in his set of tax initiatives last year, which has not yet been enacted, is an above-the-line deduction for long-term care insurance. This approach has considerable bipartisan support in Congress. Proposals have been introduced by Senator Chuck Grassley, Representative Johnson, and others, and these kinds of initiatives stand a real chance of passage for this year. The White House will continue to work with Congress to get more support for the long-term-care insurance industry, to provide a more viable option for more people as an alternative to Medicaid spend-down.

We are also pursuing other steps to help supplement private health insurance markets, such as providing better information to seniors on long-term-care needs. We are working with the U.S. Office of Personnel Management to implement a long-term-care insurance benefit shortly within the Federal Employees Health Benefit Program. These kinds of programs should provide models for additional access to good long-term-care insurance, both through employer plans and outside of employer plans. We also support some tax incentives for employer-provided coverage within cafeteria plans and the like, as well.

A lot of informal care already helps keep people out of nursing homes. This is the main source of support for people with long-term-care needs. In his budget last year, President Bush proposed a new personal exemption for persons who provide significant long-term-care assistance to family members or are caregivers in other capacities. This would provide an additional financial incentive to help seniors receive care outside of nursing homes. Bipartisan proposals similar to ours give at least respite care, some respite assistance, some additional financial assistance to the family caregivers who are providing such an important part of our long-term-care support networks.

In addition, the Administration on Aging provides a large number of programs for family caregiver support. In our budget this past year, we were able to get more than $1 billion in funding to continue these activities, and we look forward to continuing to work with Congress to strengthen and improve these programs in the next budget cycle, as well. Finally, there is a substantial shortage of various types of nursing care in this country. Last year the president proposed additional support for the education of more nurses in a wide range of nursing professions.

One part of this conference has been devoted to the coordination—or, unfortunately, the lack of coordination—of chronic care, long-term-care programs, including many of those that I have just mentioned, and acute medical services. This is a real problem, especially for older Americans. More and more medical care involves the management, often the very effective management, of chronic conditions that can lead to disabilities. When disabilities do occur in association with chronic illnesses, this management can lead to improved functional status through better support technologies and other services.

Medicare has not done a terrific job in the past of providing such integrated care, and one of the main areas of focus of the framework for Medicare legislation that the president proposed in July 2001 was improvement in the coordination of care to provide the kinds of services that many Medicare beneficiaries need today. This includes disease management services that will help seniors with chronic illnesses avoid complications from those illnesses and help them get support for those complications when they do occur and increased support for private health insurance plans and Medicare plans that have the right incentives for providing chronic care and integrated services.

The Medicare Plus Choice program today provides assistance for individuals with chronic illnesses. Medicare Plus Choice is an important option for millions of the nation's elderly and disabled, and it has helped beneficiaries get a range of benefits that are not available in the traditional Medicare program: prescription drugs, widespread use of disease management programs, supportive care, and the like.

We are now facing a major challenge in the Medicare Plus Choice program, with many plans leaving the program. Since 1998, literally hundreds of plans have left Medicare, severely reduced their service areas, or cut benefits, adversely affecting coverage for hundreds of thousands of Medicare beneficiaries. Program departures and reduction in benefits have occurred for many reasons, some of them regulatory. But there have also been problems with reimbursement. Specifically, between 1998 and 2002, Medicare Plus Choice reimbursement rates increased at only 2 to 3 percent a year, or only about 11.5 percent overall in the vast majority of counties in which Medicare Plus Choice beneficiaries live. This contrasts with increases in private health insurance premiums, which have gone up by about 15 to 18 percent a year over the past several years, and even contrasts with payment growth in the Medicare fee-for-service program, where spending over the same period increased by about 21 percent—roughly double the increase in Medicare Plus Choice payments. So it should be no surprise that these plans are having a lot of trouble continuing to offer the innovative benefits that Medicare beneficiaries prefer.

The Medicare Plus Choice payment system must be more responsive to the health-care marketplace and to the costs of providing care. At the very least it must keep better pace with increases in costs in the traditional Medicare fee-for-service payment system so that beneficiaries will continue to have access to these valuable and innovative services.

An important part of this is risk adjustment of Medicare beneficiary payments. The Centers for Medicare and Medicaid Services suspended its previous risk adjustment schedule last summer amid concerns both that it would be difficult for plans to administer (because it relied essentially on a fee-for-service structure of reporting information) and that it might not provide good incentives for chronic care and a number of chronic illnesses. The Centers for Medicare and Medicaid Services is hard at work on improving this system, and I think you can expect a proposal from them soon, moving forward with what we think will be a better risk adjustment system. It will not only give plans the financial support they need but, coupled with our other proposed changes in the

Medicare Plus Choice program, will give plans more flexibility and greater ability to provide the chronic-care and integrated-care benefits that seniors deserve.

Provision of these services is a serious problem now. Chronic-care management programs are common in private insurance plans that are available to people under age 65, yet they are rare in Medicare. Although there is certainly the capacity out there to provide these kinds of chronic-care and supportive services, they are not very widely used; only a few health maintenance organizations in the program are providing these important services.

In addition, one private plan in the program is trying to provide similar services for the sickest of the sick, the institutionalized long-term-care population. Even there, however, they are facing regulatory and financial barriers. The regulatory barriers include obstacles created by requirements for marketing that are really intended to make sure that health plans do not target the healthiest beneficiaries. The problem with strict regulations of this sort is that this plan cannot market to the nursing homes and the specific beneficiaries for whom it is particularly designed. This is a real problem in improving access to important Medicare Plus Choice services. That kind of regulatory barrier, along with the financial disincentives that I have already discussed, is an obstacle to providing good integrated care for Medicare beneficiaries that I am hopeful we can address this year in working with Congress. We really cannot wait any longer to help shore up the Medicare program.

Finally, the administration is pursuing a number of demonstration programs in Medicare related to the delivery of integrated care delivery, disease management, and the like. The president, in his framework for Medicare legislation, expressed a strong commitment to improving and building on these programs to make these kinds of services more widely available to Medicare beneficiaries. It makes good economic sense: flexible benefits are a far more cost-effective way to treat beneficiaries with chronic illnesses and disabilities than the rigid, outdated structure of benefits in the traditional Medicare plan. So, again, we hope that we can work with Congress to move forward on improving those programs as well.

We have been struggling with a number of other major health-care initiatives this year. This is an important year for health care in the United States. Not only are medical costs rising rapidly, not only are people facing problems with affordability of coverage, but we are also in the midst of a recession. Although we all hope it will soon be over, in the meantime well over a million workers have lost their jobs in just the past six months, and over the duration of the recession, more than a million and a half. Unfortunately, for many of those workers there is no available assistance with health insurance costs.

Since October, when the president first proposed that Congress enact an economic security package that could help stimulate the economy, create more jobs, and provide additional assistance to workers who have lost their jobs, we have tried to work hard with Congress to enact legislation that meets these goals; and we have gotten close. The House of Representatives has now passed two bills that provide a combination of economic stimulus and displaced-worker assistance. The bill that I want to focus on is a compromise effort that passed the House shortly before Christmas, around December 20, 2001. That bill included a bold new proposal to provide health-care assistance for displaced workers.

Under this proposal, displaced workers would get assistance with 60 percent of the cost of their health-care coverage. They could use it to continue their COBRA coverage, if they were COBRA-eligible; to continue their mini-COBRA coverage, if they were not eligible for COBRA but resided in one of the thirty-eight states that have extensions of COBRA laws that generally apply even to businesses with as few as two employees; or to continue their nongroup insurance, as about 10 or 15 percent of displaced workers had at the time that they lost their jobs. In essence, they could use it for any option that would best fit their needs.

That provision was in the House bill. It would provide assistance not only for expenses in 2002 and 2003 but also, retrospectively, for those incurred in 2001. Displaced workers would be reimbursed on their next tax returns for 60 percent of the cost of coverage while they were out of work, regardless of their income, regardless of their tax liability. This is completely refundable assistance; moreover, as it would be another unemployment benefit, it could be quickly implemented: it could be provided by the local unemployment offices, the one-stop offices that already offer an integrated set of other benefits for displaced workers, ranging from income support to training and eligibility for a hundred other programs, as well.

Assistance to displaced workers is one part of the social insurance net that has not, at least historically, been especially strong. We now have a historic opportunity to move forward, at least on a temporary basis, with a new approach. This proposal also has majority support in the Senate, and the administration is working hard now with the Senate to try to reach a compromise that would enable it to become law while it still has a chance to help workers displaced by the recent turn in the economy. On the part of the president, then, and on the part of a majority in both houses of Congress, there is a clear commitment to providing quick assistance to displaced workers with their health insurance costs.

Contributors

Maribeth Bersani is the National Director of Government Affairs at Sunrise Assisted Living.

Christine Bishop is a Professor at the Heller Graduate School, Brandeis University, and since 1979 has been a member of the research staff at the Schneider Institute for Health Policy.

David Blumenthal is Director of the Institute for Health Policy, Massachusetts General Hospital/Partners Health Care System, and Professor of Medicine and Professor of Health Care Policy at the Harvard Medical School.

Cristina Boccuti is a health policy analyst at the Urban Institute.

Richard Bringewatt is President and Chief Executive Officer of the National Chronic Care Consortium and was its cofounder and principal architect.

Benjamin Cardin has represented Maryland's Third Congressional District in the U.S. House of Representatives since 1987.

Chris Collins is a Principal with Progressive Health Partners, a health policy consulting company

John Cutler is Project Leader for the Federal Long Term Care Insurance Program at the U.S. Office of Personnel Management.

David Durenberger served as senior U.S. Senator from Minnesota from 1978 to 1995 and is now director of Citizens for Long-Term Care.

June Eichner is Senior Research Associate at the National Academy of Social Insurance.

Carroll L. Estes is Professor of Sociology at the University of California at San Francisco (UCSF).

Charles J. Fahey, a priest of the Diocese of Syracuse, N.Y., is currently a program officer for the Milbank Memorial Fund.

Judith Feder is a Professor and Dean of Policy Studies at Georgetown University's Institute for Health Care Research and Policy.

Bruce Fireman is a Biostatistician in the Division of Research at the Kaiser Permanente Medical Care Program in Oakland, California.

Robert B. Friedland is Associate Research Professor at the Institute for Health Care Research and Policy and the founding Director of the Center on an Aging Society, both at Georgetown University.

Jennie Chin Hansen is Executive Director of On Lok, the San Francisco nonprofit that pioneered the managed-care organization PACE (Program of All-Inclusive Care for the Elderly).

Michael Hash is a Principal at Health Policy Alternatives.

Catherine Hawes is a Professor in the Department of Health Policy and Management at Texas A&M and director of the Southwest Rural Health Research Center, one of six federally funded rural health research centers nationwide.

Mauro Hernandez is a doctoral student in the Department of Social and Behavioral Sciences, University of California, San Francisco.

Ruth Katz is the Deputy to the Deputy Assistant Secretary for the Office of Disability, Aging, and Long-Term Care Policy in the Office of the Assistant Secretary for Planning and Evaluation at the U.S. Department of Health and Human Services.

Marty Lynch is the Chief Executive Officer of Lifelong Medical Care, a Berkeley-based community health center organization.

Theodore R. Marmor is Professor of Public Policy and Management at the Yale School of Management and a Professor in the Department of Political Science.

Mark McClellan now directs the Food and Drug Administration and was a member of the Council of Economic Advisers.

Ingrid McDonald is responsible for policy research and legislative advocacy on behalf of the more than 120,000 members of the Service Employees International Union who work in nursing-home settings.

Mark Merlis is an independent health policy consultant in New Hope, Pennsylvania.

Marilyn Moon is a Senior Fellow in the Health Policy Center of the Urban Institute and served as Public Trustee of the Social Security and Medicare trust funds from 1995 to 2000.

John Rother is Director of Policy and Strategy at AARP.

William Scanlon is Director of Health Care Issues at the U.S. General Accounting Office.

Thomas A. Scully is the Administrator of the Centers for Medicare and Medicaid Services, responsible for the management of Medicare, Medicaid, the State Children's Health Insurance Programs, and other national health-care initiatives.

Joanne Silberner is a health policy correspondent for National Public Radio.

Deborah Stone is Research Professor of Public Policy and Government at the Rockefeller Center, Dartmouth College.

Robyn Stone is the Executive Director of the Institute on the Future of Aging Services of the American Association of Homes and Services for the Aging.

Bruce C. Vladeck is Director of the Institute for Medicare Practice and Professor of Health Policy and Geriatrics at Mount Sinai School of Medicine and Senior Vice President for Policy at Mount Sinai–New York University Health.

Mark Warshawsky is Deputy Assistant Secretary for Economic Policy at the U.S. Department of the Treasury.

Shelley I. White-Means is Professor in the Department of Economics and Research Professor in the Center for Research on Women at the University of Memphis.

Joshua M. Wiener is a Principal Research Associate at the Urban Institute, where he specializes in health policy issues.

Paul Yakoboski is Director of Policy Research for the American Council of Life Insurers.

Conference Program

National Academy of Social Insurance
14th Annual Conference

Long-Term Care and Medicare Policy:
Can We Improve the Continuity of Care?
January 24–25, 2002

Thursday, January 24, 2002

9:30	Welcome Lawrence H. Thompson, President, National Academy of Social Insurance
	Opening Speaker Benjamin Cardin, Congressman from Maryland
10:00	Session I. Chronic and Long-Term Care: What Are the Needs? Moderator: Martin Gerry, Social Security Administration
	Presenters: *Chronic and Long-Term Care Needs of Elderly and Disabled Americans* Christine Bishop, Brandeis University
	Reality of Caring for the Long-Term Care Population Robyn Stone, Institute on the Future of Aging Services

Discussants:

Paul Klaasen, Sunrise Assisted Living, Inc.

Ingrid McDonald, Service Employees International
Union

Paul Yakoboski, American Council of Life Insurers

12:00–1:15pm   Luncheon address
Thomas A. Scully, Centers for Medicare and
Medicaid Services

1:30   Session II. Care for the Elderly and Disabled under
the American Social Contract
Moderator: Marilyn Moon, Urban Institute

Presenters:
Evolution of the American Social Contract for Care
Theodore R. Marmor, Yale University

The Coverage Puzzle: How the Pieces Fit Together
Robert B. Friedland, Center on an Aging Society

The HIV-AIDS Example
Chris Collins, Progressive Health Partners

Discussants:
Michael Hash, Health Policy Alternatives, Inc.
Hunter McKay, Office of the Assistant Secretary for
Planning and Evaluation, Department of Health
and Human Services
Shelley I. White-Means, University of Memphis

3:15   Session III. Prospects for Long-Term Care
Policymaking at State and Federal Levels
Moderator: Alice Rivlin, Brookings Institution

Presenters:
David Durenberger, Citizens for Long Term Care
Judy Feder, Georgetown University
Ruth Katz, Office of Disability, Aging and Long-
Term Care Policy, Office of the Assistant
Secretary for Planning and Evaluation,
Department of Health and Human Services
Joshua M. Wiener, Urban Institute

Discussants:
John Rother, AARP

Joanne Silberner, National Public Radio

5:30–8:30   Reception and Dinner Address
                   Thomas Mann, Brookings Institution

                   2002 Heinz Dissertation Award presented by
                   Robert Hudson, Boston University, Chair of Awards
                       Committee

Friday, January 25, 2002

10:30   Session IV. Building on Experience: What Have We
                   Learned about Meeting Needs for Chronic and
                   Long-Term Care?
                   Moderator: David Blumenthal, Partners HealthCare
                       Systems

                   Presenters:
                   Bruce Fireman, Kaiser Permanente
                   Catherine Hawes, Texas A&M University
                   Marty Lynch, LifeLong Medical Care

                   Discussants:
                   Jennie Chin Hansen, On Lok
                   Bruce C. Vladeck, Mount Sinai Medical Center

12:15-1:15pm   Luncheon Speaker
                   Mark McClellan, Member, Council of Economic
                       Advisers

1:30   Session V. Visions for the Future: How Might We
                   Meet Tomorrow's Needs for Chronic and Long-Term
                   Care?
                   Moderator: Mark Warshawsky, Department of the
                       Treasury

                   Presenters:
                   Charles J. Fahey, Milbank Memorial Fund
                   Mark Merlis, Independent Health Policy Consultant
                   Deborah Stone, Dartmouth College
                   Mark Warshawsky, Department of the Treasury

                   Discussants:
                   Richard Bringewatt, National Chronic Care
                       Consortium
                   William Scanlon, General Accounting Office

Index

Page numbers followed by *f* refer to figures or tables. Page numbers followed by *n* refer to footnotes.